The
EVERYTHING®
Nutrition Book

Dear Re   healthy

We   be a

as we   ersations

major   at, and

I overl   st can't

braggi   in the gro-

help   uesday

cery   ound nutri-

night   nto the

tion i   vers each

topic   le who

nutri   book will

enjo   ormational

mak   time to

refe   give you a

tim   ating and

go

sta

The EVERYTHING® Series

Editorial

Publishing Director	Gary M. Krebs
Managing Editor	Kate McBride
Copy Chief	Laura MacLaughlin
Acquisitions Editor	Bethany Brown
Development Editor	Karen Johnson Jacot
Production Editor	Khrysti Nazzaro

Production

Production Director	Susan Beale
Production Manager	Michelle Roy Kelly
Series Designers	Daria Perreault Colleen Cunningham
Cover Design	Paul Beatrice Frank Rivera
Layout and Graphics	Colleen Cunningham Rachael Eiben Michelle Roy Kelly Daria Perreault Erin Ring
Series Cover Artist	Barry Littmann
Interior Illustrators	Argosy Publishing and Eulala Connor

Visit the entire Everything® Series at everything.com

THE
EVERYTHING
NUTRITION
BOOK

Boost energy, prevent illness,
and live longer

Kimberly A. Tessmer, R.D., L.D.

Adams Media Corporation
Avon, Massachusetts

An Everything® Series Book.
Everything® and everything.com® are registered trademarks of F+W Publications, Inc.

Published by Adams Media, an F+W Publications Company
57 Littlefield Street, Avon, MA 02322 U.S.A.
www.adamsmedia.com

ISBN: 1-58062-874-5
Printed in the United States of America.

J I H G F E D C B

Library of Congress Cataloging-in-Publication Data
Tessmer, Kimberly A.
The everything nutrition book / Kimberly A. Tessmer.
p.   cm.   (An everything series book)
ISBN 1-58062-874-5
1. Nutrition. 2. Diet. I. Title. II. Series: Everything series.
TX353 .T34 2003
613.2—dc21
2002152397

This book is available at quantity discounts for bulk purchases.
For information, call 1-800-872-5627.

Contents

11

Lightening up the Sugar / 143

12

Comprehending the Food Label / 159

13

Let's Get Cookin' / 175

14

A Healthy Start / 187

15

Nutrition to Grow With / 201

16

Nutrition Before, During, and After Pregnancy / 219

Dedication

*Special thanks to my husband, Greg,
and to my family and friends
for all of their love and support!*

Top Ten Things You'll Learn
from Reading This Book

1. How to make sense of a nutrition food label.

2. What the Food Guide Pyramid is and how it can guide you.

3. What foods belong to each food group, and how much of each you should be eating.

4. How to be a vegetarian and still meet all your nutritional needs.

5. The difference between "good" and "bad" cholesterol.

6. How to stock your kitchen and cook in ways that make the most nutritional sense.

7. The specific dietary needs for children of all ages.

8. What to eat when you are pregnant.

9. What individual vitamins and minerals do for you, and where to find the best sources of each.

10. How to tailor your nutritional intake based on your fitness level.

Introduction

▶THERE IS SO MUCH NUTRITION INFORMATION out there that includes topics such as healthy foods, nutrients, label reading, saturated fats, cholesterol, and weight loss; the list goes on and on. *The Everything® Nutrition Book* takes a look at the nutritional topics you really want to know about and provides an up-to-date comprehensive guide on each one. You will discover how healthful eating combined with physical activity promotes good health and fitness. Eating a healthy diet and maintaining a healthy weight are ways that we can help decrease our risk of health-related problems, and for most of us these issues are in our control. The more you know about nutrition, the more able you are to control your eating habits and help all those you care about. Knowledge is power! You do not need to become a nutrition expert, but you do need to understand the basics of good nutrition. This book will help you to understand the basics and provide you with the necessary information you need to maintain good health. It will provide you with practical advice on everyday eating dilemmas and challenge you to make important changes in your lifestyle, both from the nutritional and the fitness perspectives. Let this book be your guide. Use it to your advantage. Make notes in it, or jot down important information you want to remember. Don't just read this book; make it interactive. As you begin to read it, assess what goals *you* need to work on. Determine where you are currently, nutritionally, and discover what steps you need to take to improve your nutritional intake. You will find myriad tips for everything from increasing your fiber intake to decreasing your saturated fat intake. *The Everything® Nutrition Book* will even provide you with numerous nutrition and health resources to aid you in finding further information or support with certain health conditions. This book continually emphasizes that the key to good health is lifestyle change. The changes you make—whether you are trying to improve your nutritional intake, lose weight, or both—need to be permanent lifestyle changes. It is time to unlock the mystery that is nutrition and get you on the road to better health. This book will give you the knowledge you need to stick with healthful eating and physical fitness for the rest of your life.

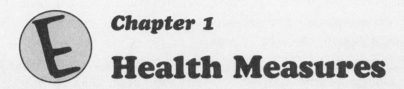

Chapter 1

Health Measures

Weight can be a major predictor of your health status. Healthy weight is a range of weight that puts you at a lower risk for chronic illnesses. Being over- or underweight places you at a higher risk for health-related problems. Maintaining a healthy weight can make it possible for you to maintain good health for a lifetime.

Weighing Your Risk

Carrying around extra weight every day can be a heavy burden to the body. Every system in the body needs to work harder. Being overweight is defined as having an excess amount of body weight that includes muscle, bone, fat, and water. Being obese specifically refers to an excess amount of body fat. Bodybuilders or athletes with a lot of muscle can be overweight without being obese. Obesity occurs when a person consumes more calories than he or she burns.

As dangerous as it is to carry around extra weight, being underweight is also associated with a higher mortality rate. Being underweight can lead to the malfunctioning of many important body functions. It can also lead to a loss of energy and an increased susceptibility to injury, infection, and illness. The causes of being either over- or underweight can be complex, and they differ among all types of individuals. Factors that include genetics, environment, social, behavioral, and psychological reasons can all add to the complexity of an abnormal body weight. You may not be able to change some of these factors, but one that you can change is your lifestyle habits.

The Health Hazards of Obesity

Losing just 5 to 10 percent of excess body weight can help to reduce your risk for health problems related to your weight. Just a small loss in body weight can help lower blood pressure, total cholesterol, LDL cholesterol (bad cholesterol), triglyceride levels, and blood sugar. Lifestyle change is the healthiest and most permanent method of losing weight and decreasing the risk for serious health problems. Combining a healthy diet with increased physical activity and behavior modification is the most successful strategy for healthy weight loss and weight maintenance.

Obesity can stress a person both physically and emotionally. Obesity can lead to feelings of low self-esteem as well as social seclusion. Since 1985, obesity has been recognized as a chronic disease. It is the second leading cause of preventable death, exceeded only by cigarette smoking. Physical health problems related to obesity include heart disease, Type 2 diabetes, high blood cholesterol levels, high blood pressure, stroke, gallbladder disease, liver disease, osteoarthritis, gout, pulmonary problems, and certain types of cancer.

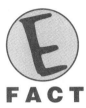

FACT

According to the National Institutes of Health (NIH), 55 percent of all adults over the age of twenty in the United States are overweight, and nearly one-quarter are obese. Obese individuals have a 50 to 100 percent increased risk of death from all causes compared with normal-weight individuals. Most of the increased risk is due to cardiovascular or heart disease.

Your Healthy Weight

The question is, are you at a healthy weight? If you are not, what is a healthy weight for you? The answer is not as easy as stepping on a scale or comparing your weight to another person's. A healthy weight is one that is right for *you,* and one that you can realistically maintain for a lifetime. Everyone is different, so even though you may be the same height, age, and gender as someone else, that does not necessarily mean you should both weigh the same.

The chart in **FIGURE 1-1** can give you a general idea of whether you are at a healthy weight.

The Healthy Weight Chart offers general guidelines for determining a reasonable weight range based on your height and weight. The higher weight in the ranges typically applies to those people who have more muscle and/or a larger body frame. People with less muscle and a smaller frame will fall at the lower end of the range. People whose weight falls above or below the specified ranges are at an increased risk of certain health conditions and disabilities.

There are many reasons that weight differs from person to person. There is no "ideal weight" or "perfect body" that everyone should attempt to shoot for. Your genetic makeup plays an important role in determining your body size and shape. Your metabolic rate, along with what you eat and your level of physical activity, also makes a considerable difference when assessing your weight.

FIGURE 1-1
Healthy Weight
Chart

Height*

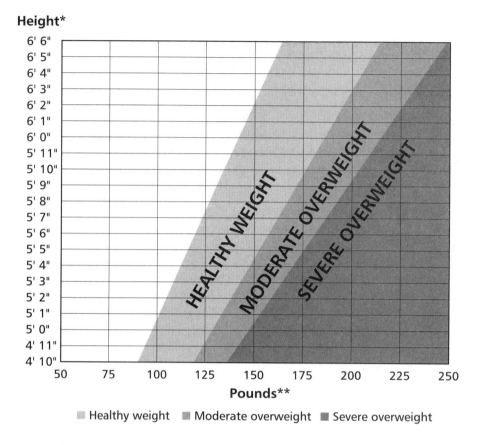

Pounds**

Healthy weight   Moderate overweight   Severe overweight

* Without shoes.
** Without clothes. The higher weights apply to people with more muscle and bone, such as many men.

Source: Report of the Dietary Guidelines Advisory Committee on the Dietary Guidelines for Americans, *1995, pages 23–24.*

Metabolic rate is defined as the rate at which your body burns energy or calories. Muscle burns more calories than fat: the more muscle your body has, the higher your metabolism will be. Your physical activity level and your age also play a role in determining your metabolic rate. Your body composition, or how much of your weight is fat, is also an important factor to consider. All of these reasons have one thing in common: they are all unique to *you.*

Assessing Your Weight

There are different factors to consider when evaluating your weight. Body weight should *not* be the only method used in assessing your weight and health. Body weight alone does not convey how much body fat you have or where it is stored—the strongest predictors of health risk. It is important to know how much of your weight is body fat, where that body fat is located, and if you already have health problems related to your weight. A number of assessment methods can be used to assess and determine whether a person is at a healthy weight. Some of these methods are based on height and weight, while others are based on measurements of body fat. The general idea is to determine whether your weight puts you at risk for health problems so that you can take action if necessary.

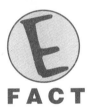

FACT

To properly weigh yourself, weigh on the same scale each time you weigh in. Use a beam balance scale, not a spring scale, whenever possible. Be sure the scale is periodically calibrated for accuracy. Wear lightweight clothing, and do not wear shoes. For consistency, try to weigh yourself at the same time of day each time. (Morning is best.)

Your body shape can be used in assessing your weight. Where you store body fat can be an indication of a healthy weight and health status. Are you an "apple" shape, storing excess body fat in the stomach area and around the waist? An apple shape can put you at higher risk for certain health problems, such as early heart disease, high blood pressure, Type 2 diabetes, and certain types of cancer. Are you a "pear" shape, storing excess body fat below the waist, in the hips, buttocks, and thighs? A pear shape does not appear to be as harmful to a person's health.

If you cannot tell by looking at your body in the mirror whether you are an apple or a pear shape, you can figure your waist-to-hip ratio. Your waist-to-hip ratio can help determine if the location of your body fat puts you at a higher risk for health-related problems. Follow these steps to figure out your waist-to-hip ratio.

1. Use a ninety-six-inch tape measure.
2. Stand relaxed. Measure your waist at its smallest point without sucking in your stomach.
3. Measure your hips by measuring the largest part of your buttocks and hips.
4. Divide your waist measurement by your hip measurement.
5. If this number is nearly or more than 1.0, you would be considered an apple shape.
6. If this number is considerably less than 1.0, you would be considered a pear shape.

Table 1-1 Where does your waist-to-hip measurement fall?		
Health Risk	**Men**	**Women**
High Risk	>1.0	>0.85
Moderately High Risk	0.90–1.0	0.80–0.85
Low Risk	<0.90	<0.80

Measuring Body Composition

Another valuable tool in assessing a healthy weight is measuring body composition, or the components that make up the structure of your body. These components include body fat and lean body mass. How much of your weight is actually body fat is one of the most significant factors in evaluating your health. For this reason, measuring body composition can be a very insightful tool.

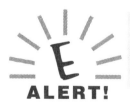

If you have more than 15 or 20 pounds to lose, have health problems, or are taking medications on a regular basis, you should see your doctor before beginning to lose weight.

Lean Body Mass vs. Body Fat

Lean body mass includes your muscle mass as well as your heart muscle, tissues of other internal organs, water, and bone. How much lean body mass you have determines your metabolism, or the rate at which your body burns calories. The higher your amount of lean body mass, the higher your metabolic rate. The higher your metabolic rate, the easier it is for you to maintain a healthy weight. You can increase lean body mass through exercise, especially strength training.

An excess of body fat is associated with chronic health problems. A bodybuilder or athlete can be overweight but not necessarily be overly fat. A person can be at a normal weight but still be carrying too much body fat. Health problems worsen as the amount of body fat increases. However, when body fat returns to within acceptable ranges, the body can return to normal healthy functioning, and the risk for developing health problems decreases.

Various methods can be used to measure body composition. Some of these methods include the hydrostatic (or underwater weighing method), bioelectrical impedance analysis (BIA), and skin-fold thickness. All methods have their pros and cons.

Hydrostatic Method

With this method, the percent body fat is calculated from equations based on the density of the body. The density of the body is calculated by measuring a person suspended on a trapeze-type scale under water. The person must exhale as much as possible. The hydrostatic method is the most accurate, but the procedure is limited to laboratories with specialized equipment and can be very expensive. This test can also be distressing, as it requires the subject to be submerged for a certain period of time.

Bioelectrical Impedance

Body fat can be measured using bioelectrical impedance analysis, or BIA. A harmless electrical current is sent through the body, measuring the resistance of body tissue. The body's ability to conduct the electrical current reflects the total amount of water in the body. The quicker the current travels, the more muscle you have. Fat stores impede the electrical current, so the slower the current, the more fat. The BIA method measures the speed and strength of the electrical current and then uses it along with information—such as age, gender, height, weight, and fitness level—to estimate the amount of body fat and lean body mass the person has.

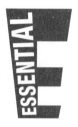

Experts recommend that you should seriously try to lose weight if you have two or more of the following: family history of certain chronic diseases, such as heart disease and diabetes; pre-existing medical conditions, such as high blood pressure, high cholesterol levels, and high blood sugar levels; and/or an apple shape or weight that is concentrated around the waist area.

It is important for the person to be properly hydrated during a BIA; otherwise, the results can be overestimated or underestimated. The BIA method can overpredict body fat in lean and athletic people unless the machine is equipped with an "athlete" mode with appropriate predictive formulas. Be aware that BIA also does not take into account the location of body fat, which again is a major predictor of health status.

Skin-Fold Thickness

The skin-fold thickness method uses a very simple caliper tool. The calipers measure subcutaneous fat (or the fat that lies just beneath the skin) of the triceps, abdomen, thighs, and chest. A pinch of the skin is pulled away from the underlying muscle, and the width of the skin is measured with the calipers. Each measurement is taken three times, and the average is taken of those measurements. These measurements are then entered into a specialized equation, and the body fat percentage is estimated. Skin-fold thickness measuring is quick and inexpensive. It takes a great deal of practice and can vary widely when measured by different examiners.

Table 1-2 Healthy Body Fat Ranges		
	Healthy Range of Body Fat	
Age	**for Females**	**for Males**
18–39	21–32 percent	8–19 percent
40–59	23–33 percent	11–21 percent
60–79	24–35 percent	13–24 percent

Source: Shape Up America, *founded by C. Everett Koop*

Body Mass Index

Body mass index, or BMI, is another tool used to determine healthy weight. BMI can inform you of the level of your health risk, given your weight and height. It can also help you realize where your weight should be to put you at the lowest risk for health problems associated with your weight. This index can provide some insight into whether you weigh more or less than you should.

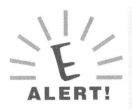

ALERT!

Be aware that BMI can misclassify as many as one in four people. It should not be used for bodybuilders, sedentary people, the elderly and/or frail, pregnant or lactating women, or growing children. BMI does give you a general idea of your health risks related to weight, but it does not distinguish between lean body mass and body fat. Many factors need to be considered when estimating how much you should weigh. Use BMI only as a general guide.

BMI uses an intricate mathematical formula based on your height and your weight. It is defined as body weight (in kilograms) divided by height (in meters squared). A high BMI can put you at an increased risk for developing certain health problems related to your weight. A healthy BMI for an adult is between 18.5 and 24.9.

To figure out your BMI, use the following equation:

1. Weight (pounds) / 2.2 = weight in kilograms (kg)
2. Height (inches) / 39.37 = height in meters (m)
3. Weight (kg) / height (m)^2 = BMI

Check your BMI against the following chart to see where your present weight places you for risk of health problems related to your body weight:

BMI	Risk for health problems related to body weight
20–25	Very low risk
26–30	Low risk
31–35	Moderate risk
36–40	High risk
40–plus	Very high risk

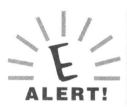
ALERT!

If your BMI is greater than 30, you should consult your personal physician for further evaluation. Health-care providers generally agree that people who have a BMI greater than 30 can improve their health greatly through weight loss.

What Are Calories?

To understand how to achieve and maintain a healthy weight, you need to start with your calorie needs. It is possible to manage your weight by balancing the calories you eat and the physical activities you choose. Calories measure the amount of energy in foods. Your body relies on calories to keep you alive and moving.

There are three nutrients in foods that provide calories, or energy.

These three nutrients include carbohydrates, protein, and fat. These nutrients are released from food during the digestive process and then absorbed into the bloodstream and converted to glucose or blood sugar. Glucose is your body's main source of energy.

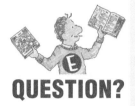

QUESTION?

How many calories do nutrients provide?
Carbohydrates, protein, and fat are the *only* three nutrients that provide calories in food. Fat provides 9 calories per gram, carbohydrates provide 4 calories per gram, and protein provides 4 calories per gram.

Your Body's Calorie Needs

Your body constantly needs calories or energy. Having a general idea of your body's total calorie needs can help you to maintain, lose, or gain weight. Everyone's caloric needs differ, depending on factors such as age, gender, size, body composition, basal metabolic rate, and physical activity.

Basal metabolic rate (BMR) is the rate at which your body burns calories when at rest. It is the level of energy your body needs to keep your normal body processes going, such as heartbeat, breathing, keeping your body temperature regulated, and transmitting messages to your brain. Your BMR uses up 60 percent of your body's total energy needs.

Estimating Your Calorie Needs

There are different methods for estimating caloric needs for individuals. Though just an estimate, it can give you a general idea of the amount of calories your body needs. Whether you are overweight, at your healthy weight, or underweight, it is important to be aware of the calories you should be consuming for good health and to reach or maintain a healthy weight. The following is a simple equation that can help you easily estimate your caloric needs:

1. Figure your BMR by multiplying your healthy weight (in pounds) by 10 for women and 11 for men. If you are overweight, use the average

weight within the range given on the Healthy Weight Chart (**FIGURE 1-1**). Using your actual weight, if you are overweight, will overestimate your calorie needs.

2. Figure your calorie needs for physical activity. Multiply your BMR, from step 1, by the percentage that matches your activity level: sedentary, 20 percent; light activity, 30 percent; moderate activity, 40 percent; very active, 50 percent.

3. Add calories needed for digestion and absorption of nutrients in your body. Add your calories for BMR, from step 1, and your calories for physical activity, from step 2, then multiply the total by 10 percent.

4. Add up your total calorie needs by adding the calories from each step.

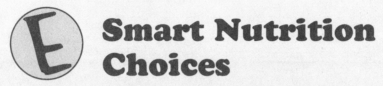

Chapter 2

Smart Nutrition Choices

Eating is one of our simplest and greatest pleasures. Eating a healthy diet does not have to be a difficult task. Healthy eating is made easier by following simple dietary guidelines that provide a general outline of what to eat each day. Making smart nutrition choices and adopting healthy lifestyle habits is the key to good health.

The Dietary Guidelines

The U.S. Department of Agriculture (USDA) and the U.S. Department of Health and Human Services (HHS) created the Dietary Guidelines for Americans 2000. These guidelines were designed to help people know what to eat to stay healthy. They reflect the most up-to-date and sound nutrition information known about healthy eating and a healthy lifestyle. The guidelines provide the best nutrition advice about choosing and preparing foods, as well as about living an active lifestyle that will help promote health and prevent disease. The Dietary Guidelines for Americans apply to all healthy Americans over the age of two. The guidelines include ten specific guidelines that carry three basic messages: aim for fitness, build a healthy base, and choose sensibly.

Aim for Fitness

The first message of the Dietary Guidelines for Americans is to aim for fitness. This aim includes both a healthy weight and regular physical activity. Regular physical activity will help you reach and/or maintain your healthy weight. Following these first two guidelines will help keep you productive and feeling your best.

Aim for a Healthy Weight

As discussed in Chapter 1, it is important to evaluate your body weight and to know if you are at a healthy weight or what your healthy weight should be. If you need to lose weight, it is recommended to lose gradually. A loss of ½ to 2 pounds per week is an acceptable and safe level of weight loss. If you are at a healthy weight, your goal should be to prevent further weight gain. Being obese or overweight increases your risk for many health problems. A healthy weight is an important key to a long and healthy life.

Be Physically Active Each Day

In addition to maintaining a healthy weight, physical activity is essential to good health. Adults should try for at least thirty minutes of moderate physical activity most days of the week. Choose activities that you enjoy and can realistically do on a regular basis. If you already get thirty minutes of activity daily, you can benefit your health by either increasing the amount of time you exercise or increasing the intensity. In addition to being essential for good health, regular physical activity is essential to losing weight and/or maintaining your healthy weight.

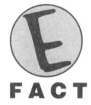

FACT

Moderate physical activity is defined as any activity that requires about as much energy as walking two miles in thirty minutes.

It is most beneficial to include aerobic activity, flexibility, and strength training to your regular exercise routine. Regular physical activity is important, but being more active in your daily routine can also benefit your health. Doing everyday activities can add to your day's total of moderate activity. Ways to add more daily physical activity include the following:

- Take the stairs instead of the elevator or escalator.
- Park farther away from the building for a longer walk.
- Wash the car yourself instead of taking it to the car wash.
- Skip the drive-through at the bank and walk in instead.
- Use a restroom at work that is on another floor or at the other end of the building.
- Get up twenty minutes earlier in the morning and start your day with a brisk walk.
- Walk the dog to make sure she/he gets exercise too!
- Don't just watch your kids play; get out there and play with them.

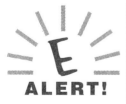

ALERT!

If you have chronic health problems, are on medication, are currently seeing your health-care provider for a specific health problem, are at high risk for heart disease, or are over the age of 40 for men and 50 for women, you should consult your health-care provider before starting any exercise plan.

Build a Healthy Base

These next four guidelines will help you build a healthy base to your diet. Forming a solid base is crucial because it is what the rest of your diet is built on. Letting the Food Guide Pyramid help build your base as well as the rest of your diet will ensure a healthy and well-balanced eating plan.

Let the Pyramid Guide Your Food Choices

The Food Guide Pyramid can help you make healthy food choices, providing all the nutrients necessary for good nutrition and good health. The pyramid shape is designed to show you what you should eat the most of—in the base, or largest part of the pyramid—and what you should eat the least of at the tip, or smallest part of the pyramid. Your basic eating pattern should be built on the foundation of plant foods (the base of the pyramid, or the bottom three blocks) that include fruits, vegetables, and grains. Next, you should include low-fat or fat-free dairy products and lean foods from the meat and bean group each day (the next two blocks of the pyramid). The tip of the pyramid contains foods you should eat the least of, sweets and fats.

Choose a Variety of Grains Daily

Foods made from grains should be the base of a nutritious diet. Grains include bread, rice, pasta, and oats. Refined grains differ from whole grains. Refined grains include white bread and white rice. Refined grains are much lower in important nutrients, so you should choose whole grains more often.

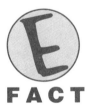

FACT

Refined grains are made from white flour. White flour is made only from the endosperm of the grain. The endosperm has most of the protein and carbohydrate but has smaller amounts of nutrients such as vitamins, minerals, and fiber. Whole-grain or whole-wheat products are made from 100 percent whole-wheat flour, including the bran, endosperm, and germ.

When choosing grains, look for the words "whole grain" or "whole wheat" to make sure the product is made from 100 percent whole-wheat flour. Whole-grain foods are packed with vitamins, minerals, fiber, and complex carbohydrates. These foods are usually low in fat unless fat is added in processing or preparation. The aim should be to consume at least six servings of grain products per day. Choose grains that are rich in fiber, low in saturated fat, and low in sodium.

Choose a Variety of Fruits and Vegetables Daily

Eating a variety of fruits and vegetables is key to a healthy diet. Fruits and vegetables are rich in different essential nutrients such as vitamins, minerals, and fiber. Eating a variety ensures a greater intake of these essential nutrients. Aim to try different types and colors. Whether you are choosing fresh, frozen, canned, dried, or juice, you will receive the added benefits of this healthy food group. Juices and canned fruits do not provide as much fiber as the other types, so it is best to choose the others more often. Eat at least five servings per day of fruits and vegetables, consisting of at least two servings of fruit and three servings of vegetables.

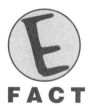

FACT

Research by the American Institute for Cancer suggests that people aim for meals composed of two-thirds (or more) plant-based foods like vegetables, fruits, whole grains, and beans, and one-third (or less) animal protein.

Keep Food Safe

It is as important to eat healthy foods as it is to keep the foods you eat safe from harmful bacteria, parasites, and viruses. "Safe" means you are taking the necessary steps to decrease the risk of foodborne illnesses from eating contaminated food. People at higher risk for foodborne illness include pregnant women, young children, older persons, and people with weakened immune systems.

Some common causes of foodborne illnesses include salmonella, staphylococcus aureus, E. coli, and clostridium perfringens. To keep your food safe, wash your hands and work surfaces often; separate raw, cooked, and ready-to-eat food when you shop for, cook, or store foods; cook foods to safe temperatures; chill perishable foods promptly; follow the safety instructions on labels; keep hot foods hot and cold foods cold; and when in doubt throw it out.

People who have a higher risk of foodborne illnesses should take extra precautions:

- Do not eat or drink unpasteurized juices, raw sprouts, raw or unpasteurized milk, or products made from unpasteurized milk.
- Do not eat raw or undercooked meat, poultry, eggs, fish, or shellfish such as clams, oysters, scallops, and mussels.

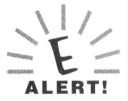

ALERT!

The danger zone for foods is between 40 and 140 degrees Fahrenheit. In this range, bacteria grow the quickest and can produce toxins causing foodborne illness. To be safe when cooking meat, be sure to cook the meat to the correct internal temperature. Use a meat thermometer. Make sure ground meat products are cooked to at least 160 degrees; roasts and steak are cooked to at least 145 degrees; pork is cooked to at least 160 degrees; and poultry is cooked to at least 170 degrees.

Choose Sensibly

Making sensible and healthy food choices can promote health and can even help reduce your risk for some chronic diseases. All foods can be part of a healthy diet if you don't overdo it on nutrients such as sodium, fat, saturated fat, sugar, and alcohol. The key to enjoying a healthy diet is eating in moderation.

Choose a Diet Low in Saturated Fat and Cholesterol and Moderate in Total Fat

Fats are an essential part of a healthy diet. They supply energy and essential fatty acids and help fat-soluble vitamins (A, D, E, and K) to absorb in the body. The key is choosing foods sensibly that will not provide too much fat or the wrong type of fat. Eating too much fat, no matter what type it is, will add excess calories to your diet.

There are various types of fat, which include saturated and unsaturated fats. Saturated fats can increase the risk for coronary heart disease by raising blood cholesterol. Saturated fats are found mainly in animal foods. Unsaturated fat does not increase blood cholesterol and can even help to lower it. Unsaturated fats are found mainly in vegetable and fish oils. Dietary cholesterol is different from dietary fat. Cholesterol is a fatlike substance but is not fat itself. Cholesterol has different functions than fat in the body and has a different structure than fat. The body does need some cholesterol for normal function, but too much cholesterol has been linked to heart disease.

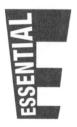

The aim is to limit solid fats, such as butter or lard, because they are higher in saturated fats. Use vegetable oils instead. When consuming dairy products, choose low-fat or fat-free products. Choose lean meats, fish, poultry, and dried beans as protein sources.

Choose Beverages and Foods to Moderate Your Intake of Sugars

Sugars are simple carbohydrates that the body uses as a source of energy. During digestion, all carbohydrates break down into sugar, or blood glucose. Some sugars occur naturally, such as in dairy products (as lactose) and fruits (as fructose). Other foods have added sugars, or sugar that is added in processing or preparation. The body cannot tell the difference between naturally occurring sugar and added sugar. Most foods containing added sugars provide calories but little in the way of essential nutrients such as fiber, vitamins, and minerals.

Food containing added sugar can also promote tooth decay. Major sources include soft drinks, drinks such as fruit punch or lemonade, cakes, cookies, pies, dairy desserts such as ice cream, and candy. The aim is to get most of your calories from grains, fruits, vegetables, low-fat or fat-free dairy products, and lean meats and/or meat substitutes. Don't let sugary beverages such as soft drinks replace more nutritious beverages such as milk, juice, or water. Sugar can be part of a healthy diet if consumed in moderation.

Choose and Prepare Foods with Less Salt

Consuming less salt can reduce your risk for developing high blood pressure. Eating less salt can also contribute to a decrease in the loss of bone calcium. Sodium and salt are *not* the same thing. Table salt is the common name for sodium chloride. Table salt is 40 percent sodium and 60 percent chloride. Consuming too much sodium can have negative impacts on health, but sodium also has many essential functions in the body. The problem is that most people consume too much.

Only small amounts of salt occur naturally in foods. Most of the salt people consume is added during food processing, during preparation in a restaurant or at home, or at the table. The aim should be for a moderate sodium intake. Healthy adults need to consume only small amounts of salt to meet the body's sodium needs.

If You Drink Alcoholic Beverages, Do So in Moderation

Alcoholic beverages supply plenty of calories and very few nutrients. Alcohol can be harmful when consumed in excess. More than one drink per day for women or two drinks per day for men can raise the risk for high blood pressure, stroke, and certain types of cancer. Heavy drinkers are at risk for malnutrition because alcohol contains calories that may substitute for those in nutritious foods. If adults drink alcohol, they should do so in moderation and with meals to slow the absorption of the alcohol. Moderation is defined as no more than one drink per day for women and no more than two drinks per day for men.

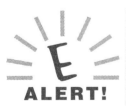
ALERT!

The health risks associated with increased alcohol consumption include high blood pressure, obesity, and stroke. At this time, no clinical trials have been performed to test the alcohol-CHD (Coronary Heart Disease) relation. If you're a heavy drinker, statistics show that cutting back can help reduce your risk for stroke.

What Is the Food Guide Pyramid?

In 1992, the USDA developed the Food Guide Pyramid. The Food Guide Pyramid goes beyond the basic food groups to help put the Dietary Guidelines for Americans into action. The pyramid contains the building blocks essential to a healthy diet. It gives the guidance you need to recognize what and how much to eat of each of five major food groups daily. Following the Food Guide Pyramid will help you keep your fat intake at recommended levels and help you consume all the essential nutrients that make up a healthy diet.

Keys to the Pyramid

The pyramid conveys three messages: variety, balance, and moderation. Eating a variety of foods within each group ensures that you meet your nutritional requirements and also provides a much wider variety of nutrients to your diet. Variety can make eating more interesting, a lot more fun, and more palatable. A healthy eating plan should be designed around the foods you like to eat. Keep your total calorie count in line with your weight loss or weight maintenance goals.

Balance means eating from all the food groups and balancing them out each day. Don't eat all of your calories just from one food group and forget about the others. Balancing the food groups in your diet provides variety and supplies a better balance of nutrients.

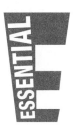

To add variety to your daily diet, you might try new recipes (swap recipes with friends and family), try a new cookbook (check out your local library so you can try many of them), or go to the grocery store and notice all of the fruits and vegetables you have never tried. Choose a new one each week to buy and try!

To eat in moderation, choose the number of servings that meet your calorie needs and try to control the total amount of fat, cholesterol, sodium, sugar, and alcoholic beverages you consume. There is a place in a healthy diet for all types of foods. Eating higher fat and/or higher sugar foods is part of a realistic eating plan as long as you eat them in moderation and refrain from overindulging. Don't forget that the tip of the pyramid is fat and sugar—you should *limit* them, not avoid them.

Inside the Food Guide Pyramid

The food groups in the pyramid include the following:

- Breads, cereal, rice, and pasta
- Vegetables
- Fruits
- Milk, yogurt, and cheese
- Meat, poultry, fish, dry beans, eggs, nuts, and meat substitutes
- Sweets and fats

Foods in one food group should not replace foods from another food group. One food group is not more important than another. Each group supplies different essential nutrients, so it is important to eat from all of the food groups for good health. One food group alone cannot supply all of the nutrients and healthful substances that are necessary for optimal health. The Food Guide Pyramid emphasizes eating a variety of food from all of the food groups each day. The pyramid actually shows six blocks. The tip of the pyramid is the fat and sweets group. Fat is an important nutrient, but it should be eaten in moderation.

Serving Sizes

The pyramid provides a suggested range of the number of servings per food group that you should eat each day. The number of servings and the size of the servings you eat compose your daily caloric intake. Chapter 3 discusses each food group in further detail, including what constitutes a serving in each food group.

Keep in mind that serving sizes are only approximations. If you do not have any idea of what a serving size should look like, it would be a good idea to start out by measuring your foods. Once you have an idea of what they should look like, it will be easier to eye your portion sizes in the future. For mixed foods, such as pizza, do your best to estimate the food group servings contained in the food. For example, a slice of pizza can be counted as the grain group for the crust, the milk group for the cheese, and the vegetable group for the tomato sauce. If you add other toppings, such as Canadian bacon, that would count as a meat. Mushrooms would count in the vegetable group.

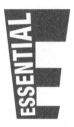

If you are a vegetarian, you can still make the Food Guide Pyramid work for you. A vegetarian who completely avoids meat, poultry, and fish can choose alternate foods from the meat group. Some of these alternate choices include peanut butter, dry beans or peas, eggs, nuts, and soy foods such as tofu, tempeh, veggie burgers, and soy milk. Use peanut butter and nuts sparingly because they tend to be high in fat.

Number of Servings

The pyramid provides a range of servings for each food group. The number of servings that is right for you depends on how many calories you need. How many calories you need depends on factors such as age, gender, weight, and how active you are. Just about everyone should have at least the minimum number of servings in each food group. The minimum number of servings adds up to about 1,600 calories. The middle number adds up to about 2,200 calories, and the maximum number of servings adds up to about 2,800 calories.

Once you know the number of calories you need each day, you can figure out the number of servings you should eat from all of the food groups. **TABLE 2-1** tells you how many servings you need for your calorie level.

Table 2-1 Servings Needed Per Calorie Level			
Food Group	**1,600**	**2,200**	**2,800**
Grains group servings	6	9	11
Vegetable group servings	3	4	5
Fruit group servings	2	3	4
Milk group servings	2–3*	2–3*	2–3*
Meat group servings (ounces)	5	6	7

*Women who are pregnant or breastfeeding, teenagers, and young adults to age twenty-four need three servings of the milk group per day.

Knowing how many servings of each food group and the size of the servings will help you to easily follow your caloric level. Don't make yourself crazy trying to count calories for each food you eat. Instead, focus on eating the number of servings for each food group that is right for you and eating healthy foods in moderation. Ⓔ

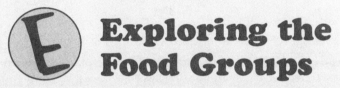

Chapter 3

Exploring the Food Groups

Besides the wonderful aromas, flavors, and textures that food has, each food group provides varying amounts of diverse nutrients. Each one of the five food groups supplies some, but not all, of the nutrients you need for good health. For this reason it's key that you eat from each food groups every day.

Bread, Cereal, Rice, and Pasta Group

The base of the Food Guide Pyramid includes all foods made from grains. These foods should form the base of a nutritious diet. Foods in the bread, cereal, rice, and pasta group—or the starch group—are rich in complex carbohydrates (or starches). Complex carbohydrates are an excellent source of energy. They are low in fat and cholesterol and are your body's main source of energy.

Health experts agree that you should consume at least half of your total daily calories from carbohydrates, especially complex carbohydrates. The Food Guide Pyramid suggests consuming six to eleven servings from the starch group each day. This may seem like a lot, but servings add up quicker than you realize, so keep serving sizes in mind.

One serving equals any of the following:

- One slice enriched or whole-grain bread
- ½ medium bagel
- One 6-inch tortilla
- ½ cup cooked rice or pasta
- ½ cup cooked oatmeal or cream of wheat
- ¾ cup ready-to-eat cereal

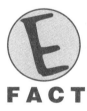

FACT

The U.S. Food and Drug Administration (FDA) now requires that enriched, refined grain products (such as breads, flours, corn-meals, rice, noodles, macaroni, and other grain products) be fortified with folic acid, a form of folate. Folate is a B vitamin that has been found to reduce the incidence of certain neural-tube birth defects in newborn babies. Whole-grain foods naturally contain some folate.

Grain foods, especially whole grains, supply vitamin E and B vitamins such as folic acid as well as minerals like magnesium, iron, and zinc. Whole grains (like whole wheat) are rich in fiber and higher in other important nutrients. In fact, eating plenty of whole grain breads, bran cereals, and other whole-grain foods can easily provide half of your fiber needs for an entire day. Eating whole grains provides you with more vitamins, minerals, fiber, phytoestrogens, lignans, antioxidants, and other protective substances that you lose when grains are refined. Whole grains add more flavor and texture to foods. When consuming your needed number of servings from the starch group, aim to get at least three servings from a whole-grain source.

Whole Grains vs. Refined Grains

Whole grains are more nutritious and wholesome than refined grains. Whole grain is the entire edible part of any grain, including wheat, corn, oats, and rice. Refined grains go through a milling process in which parts of the grain are removed. Refined grains, such as white rice or white bread, are low in fiber and other important nutrients. In refined grains, many of the essential nutrients are lost in processing. Some nutrients are added back, or the product is enriched, but this usually does not include all of the nutrients that were lost. To increase your intake of whole-grain foods, look for words such as whole grain, whole wheat, rye, bulgur, brown rice, oatmeal, whole oats, pearl barley, and whole-grain corn as one of the first words in the ingredient list on a food label.

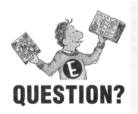

QUESTION?

What is the difference between "fortified" and "enriched"? Fortified means that nutrients are added that were not presently found in the food. For example, some varieties of orange juice are fortified with calcium. Enriched means that nutrients that originally belonged to the food were added back. These are nutrients that may have been lost in processing. When a grain product is enriched, B vitamins such as thiamine, riboflavin, niacin, and folic acid are added back to the refined grain.

Smart Starch Choices

The Food Guide Pyramid suggests building a healthy base by making a variety of grain foods the foundation of your diet. To get the most out of this important food group, follow some of the following tips.

- Choose breads, cereals, and pastas made from whole wheat or whole grain more often. Rye and pumpernickel breads are also high in fiber.
- Look for the words "high in fiber" or "good source of fiber" on food labels.
- Look for breads, rolls, and muffins with 3 grams of fat or less per serving.
- Try new foods in the grain group such as quinoa, millet, or couscous.
- Try grains in your salads by adding pastas, rice, or bulgur (as in tabouli).
- Look for the word "whole" in front of grains such as barley, corn, oats, rice, or wheat.
- Choose brown rice more often than white. Brown rice is the only type of whole-grain rice.
- Look for varieties of cereal that offer at least 3 grams of fiber, have 3 grams of fat or less, and that include 8 grams or less of sugar per serving.
- Choose breads, crackers, and crunchy snacks with less fat and sugar.

Vegetable Group

Vegetables are tasty and crunchy, and they can add lots of color and flavor to your meals. Vegetables are naturally low in calories. They have little to no fat, are cholesterol free, and are packed with fiber. Vegetables are loaded with many essential nutrients that vary greatly from one variety to the next. Eating a variety of colors and types ensures a better intake of all these nutrients.

The Food Guide Pyramid suggests consuming three to five servings from the vegetable group each day.

One serving equals any of the following:

- ½ cup chopped raw, non-leafy vegetables
- ½ cup cooked vegetables
- ¾ cup vegetable juice
- 1 cup leafy, raw vegetables
- One small baked potato (3 ounces)
- ½ cup cooked legumes (beans, peas, or lentils)

Vegetables are packed with all types of healthy nutrients. See Appendix B for more information on specific vegetables and their nutrients. Daily requirements for several vitamins—including vitamin C, folic acid, and beta-carotene, the precursor for vitamin A—can be met almost exclusively from fresh vegetables and fruits. This is especially true with dark-green leafy vegetables, such as spinach or broccoli, and dark orange vegetables, such as carrots or yams. Some vegetables also supply sufficient amounts of calcium, iron, and magnesium. In addition to nutrients, vegetables also contain compounds called phytochemicals that may provide additional health benefits.

Uncovering Phytochemicals

Phytochemicals, sometimes referred to as plant nutrients or plant chemicals, are found only in plants. Plants naturally produce these chemicals to help protect themselves against bacteria, fungi, and viruses. Phytochemicals are being researched for their health-promoting potential. Though their role is still uncertain, certain phytochemicals may help protect against illnesses such as heart disease, certain cancers, and other chronic health conditions.

Phytochemicals are found in vegetables (including cruciferous vegetables), fruits, grains, legumes, seeds, and soy. There are believed to be close to 12,000 different types of phytochemicals in plants. Some of these include lutein, lycopene, carotenoids, flavonoids, indoles, and isoflavones. The more colorful a vegetable is, the higher its phytochemical content.

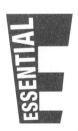

Cruciferous vegetables are members of the cabbage family, such as arugula, bok choy, broccoli, Brussels sprouts, cabbage, cauliflower, collards, kale, mustard greens, radishes, rutabaga, turnip, turnip greens, and watercress. Though the precise reasons are unclear, studies suggest that these vegetables may have properties for fighting colon and rectal cancers. You should aim to eat cruciferous vegetables several times per week.

Handle Vegetables with Care

Vegetables can be very fragile and need to be handled with care when storing, preparing, and cooking. It is important to handle vegetables with care to preserve their valuable vitamin content.

Tips for storing vegetables correctly include the following:

- Vegetables should be kept chilled (except tomatoes and potatoes).
- Store cut or peeled vegetables in the refrigerator.
- Vegetables are perishable, even if you store them properly, so buy only what you need. The freshest vegetables contain the most nutrients.
- Damage and bruising can speed up spoilage of the produce.

Tips for preparing vegetables include the following:

- Wash produce to remove any dirt and bacteria on the surface. Wash produce by rinsing in cool water, and if the surface is firm, scrubbing with a small, soft-bristled brush.
- Wash your hands before and after handling produce.
- When cutting vegetables, use a clean cutting board that is not used for other foods, such as meat.
- Trim only the inedible parts of the vegetable. Many of the nutrients found in vegetables are located in the outer leaves, in the skin, and just below the skin.

Tips for cooking vegetables include the following:

- Eat vegetables raw or cook them quickly until tender-crisp. Some vitamins, such as B vitamins and vitamin C, are very sensitive to heat and can be destroyed easily.
- Cook vegetables in a very small amount of water. Steam or microwave to preserve as much nutrient content as possible.
- Cover the pot when cooking vegetables to keep in steam and reduce cooking time.
- For vegetables that need to be cooked longer, cut in larger pieces. This will expose less of the surface and ensure that fewer vitamins are lost.

Eat Your Veggies

The best choices for vegetables are fresh, frozen, or juices. Whole vegetables are more filling and contain more fiber than vegetable juices, so choose whole vegetables more often. Canned vegetables tend to be high in sodium and lower in nutrients such as fiber. The key is to eat a variety of vegetables to supply your body with all their beneficial nutrients.

Follow these tips to help include vegetables in your daily diet:

- Keep vegetables in the house. If they're not there, chances are you won't eat them!
- Add or increase vegetables in soups, stews, and casseroles.
- Have vegetables cut up, cleaned, and stored in the refrigerator so when you have that snack attack they are easily available.
- If you don't like plain vegetables, try dipping them in fat-free dressing, adding low-fat or fat-free cheese, or adding toasted almonds or other nuts.
- Zip up recipes by adding shredded vegetables to some of your dishes, such as shredded carrots or zucchini to meatloaf, burgers, or lasagna.
- Make vegetables the focus of your meal.
- Serve more than one type of vegetable at lunch or dinner. Two is always better than one!
- Go crazy with pizza toppings by adding broccoli, shredded carrots, zucchini, peppers, or chopped tomatoes.
- Drink vegetable juice with meals or as a quick nutritious snack.

Fruit Group

Although they are not grouped together, the fruit and vegetable groups share a tier on the Food Guide Pyramid. Neither group is more important than the other, so you should eat servings from both groups. The fruit group is filled with colorful, nutritious, and delicious varieties. Most fruits have no fat, and all are cholesterol free. Fruits are loaded with many essential nutrients that vary among the varieties. Eating different fruits ensures a better intake of all the nutrients that they provide. Try as many colors and types as you can for variety.

The Food Guide Pyramid suggests consuming two to four servings from the fruit group each day.

One serving equals any of the following:

- One small to medium fresh fruit
- ½ cup canned or cut-up fresh fruit
- ¾ cup fruit juice
- ¼ cup dried fruit

Fruit's sweet flavor comes from fructose, a naturally occurring sugar. Fructose is a carbohydrate, which is a good source of energy or blood glucose and your body's main source of energy. Chapter 11 discusses sugar in more detail. Fruit is full of healthy substances such as vitamin C, vitamin A, potassium, folic acid, antioxidants, phytochemicals, and fiber, just to name a few. See Appendix B for more information on specific fruits and their nutrients. Citrus fruits, berries, and melons are excellent sources of vitamin C. Dried fruits are available all year long and are an excellent source of many nutrients including fiber.

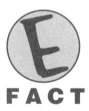

FACT

Antioxidants include beta-carotene, vitamins C and E, and some minerals such as selenium, copper, zinc, and manganese. Antioxidants help to counteract the effects of dangerous free radicals in the body that are formed by normal body processes and environmental factors. Free radicals damage body cells and tissues. This damage can lead to the onset of health problems such as cancer, heart disease, cataracts, arthritis, and other health issues that come with age. Eating a variety of fruits and vegetables ensures an adequate intake of antioxidants.

Handle Fruit with Care

Just like vegetables, it is important to handle and choose your fruits wisely for optimal nutrient content. Following certain tips can help you get the most out of the fruit group.

Tips for storing fruit include the following:

- Keep in mind that fruits are perishable, even if you store them properly, so only buy amounts you need. The freshest fruits contain the most nutrients.
- Store your fruits properly to maintain quality. Store them so you use the ripest ones first.

Tips for preparing fruits include the following:

- Wash produce to remove surface dirt and bacteria. Rinse in cool water, and if the surface is firm, scrub with a small, soft-bristled brush.
- Wash your hands before and after handling your produce.
- When cutting fruits, use a clean cutting board that is not used for other foods, such as meat.
- Leave the edible skin on fruits whenever possible. Most of the vitamins and minerals are found in the skin and in the area just below the skin.

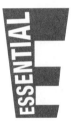

Fruits to buy and eat within a few days include these: apples, oranges, grapes, pineapple, cherries, strawberries, and watermelon. Fruits that will continue to ripen and still maintain their nutritional quality include apricots, cantaloupe, bananas, plums, peaches, pears, and nectarines.

Eat Your Fruits

Fruits offer a refreshing, crunchy, and sweet food option. The best choices for fruits are fresh, frozen, canned, dried, or fruit juices. Whole fruit is more filling and contains more fiber than fruit juices, so choose whole fruits more often. When choosing canned fruits, look for varieties that are canned in their own juice or whose labels specify "extra light syrup." The key is to eat a variety to supply your body with all fruit's nutrients.

Follow these tips to help include fruit in your daily diet:

- Keep fruit in the house. If it's not there, chances are you won't eat it!
- Look for dried fruits in the produce section. They are nonperishable and packed with nutrition and fiber.

- Eat a piece of fruit at breakfast. Cut up fruit to put in your cereal or favorite yogurt.
- If you don't have time for a piece of fruit, grab a glass of fruit juice.
- Bring a piece of fruit to work to enjoy on break or at lunch.
- Cut up fruit and have it cleaned and stored in the refrigerator so when you have that snack attack, you have some easily available.
- Try fruit for dessert.
- Try a quick and easy fruit smoothie by blending a cup of berries (or your favorite fruit) with a half cup of vanilla low-fat yogurt and a cup of ice.

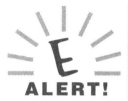

ALERT!

Some dried fruits may be preserved in sulfites. Sulfites can trigger allergic reactions in some people. If you know you have an allergy, read the ingredient labels on dried fruits to find out if sulfites are present.

The Juice Debate

When choosing fruit juices, check the label. Actual fruit juice contains fructose, the naturally occurring sugar in fruit. Fruit drinks, fruit cocktails, and fruitades contain fructose plus added sugar. When the label states "100 Percent Fruit Juice," the juice only has the naturally occurring sugar fructose and no added sugar. The body uses all sugar the same, but juice with added sugar contains more calories. The percentage of juice has nothing to do with the nutrient content, such as vitamin C, so the best advice is to check out the food label!

The Meat Group

The next tier of the Food Guide Pyramid, level three from the bottom, is the meat group. This group includes a variety of foods, including beef, pork, chicken, turkey, fish, game, eggs, dry beans (legumes, lentils, and peas), soy foods, nuts, and peanut butter. The meat group supplies large amounts of protein as well as other essential nutrients. Some of the choices in the meat group, such as nuts, dry beans, and soy foods, are plant foods. These foods are grouped with meat because they are excellent sources of protein.

You need fewer servings from the meat group because it is higher in fat. The Food Guide Pyramid suggests consuming two to three servings or about 5 to 7 ounces from the meat group each day.

One serving equals any of the following:

- 2 to 3 ounces cooked lean meat, poultry, or fish; the following count as an ounce of meat:
  - 1 egg
  - $^1/_2$ cup cooked legumes (lentils, peas, or dried beans)
  - $^1/_4$ cup egg substitute
  - 2 tablespoons peanut butter
  - $^1/_3$ cup nuts
  - 4 ounces tofu
  - 1 cup soy milk
- 2 to 3 ounces canned tuna or salmon, packed in water

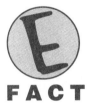

FACT

Although eggs can be a great source of protein, they are also high in dietary cholesterol. You should limit your use of whole eggs or egg yolks to no more than four per week. The only part of the egg that contains cholesterol is the egg yolk. In place of whole eggs, try using egg substitutes or egg whites, both of which are cholesterol free.

The meat group supplies varying amounts of nutrients, including zinc, iron, and B vitamins (thiamine, niacin, vitamin B_6, and vitamin B_{12}). Beef, poultry, and fish are some of the best sources of iron. These foods contain "heme" iron, which is better absorbed in the body, as opposed to the non-heme iron in plant foods. The meat group is also a source of dietary fat. The fat found in animal foods is saturated fat. Too much saturated fat in the diet can lead to increased blood cholesterol as well as heart disease.

Making Healthy Choices

The meat group is an important food group because of the nutrients it provides. However, because the majority of foods in the meat group contain saturated fat and cholesterol, it is important to make lean and low-fat choices.

Follow these tips to help make low-fat choices from the meat group:

- Choose skinless, white meat poultry.
- Instead of ground beef, try lean ground turkey instead. Ground turkey breast can be up to 99 percent fat-free.
- Buy meat that is well trimmed, with no more than an eighth of an inch fat trim. (Trim refers to the fat layer surrounding the cut of meat.)
- When buying ground meats, look for packages that have the greatest percent lean-to-fat ratio.
- When buying beef, be aware of grades and inspection of meat.
- Choose beans, peas, lentils, and soy foods often, and try to make them your main meal several times per week.
- Limit your intake of high-fat processed meats, including bacon, sausage, bologna, salami, kielbasa, bratwurst, and other higher-fat meats.
- Limit your intake of liver and other organ meats that tend to be very high in cholesterol.
- Use egg yolks and whole eggs in moderation.
- Watch your portion sizes. Three ounces of cooked meat is about the size of a deck of cards.

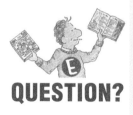

QUESTION?

What do the different grades of meat mean?
Food grades of meat are determined by the U.S. Department of Agriculture and are based on fat content, appearance, texture, and the age of the animal. The Select grade has the least marbled fat, followed by Choice cuts, then Prime. Prime cuts are the juiciest and most favorable but contain the most fat. With proper cooking techniques, Select and Choice cuts can be just as tender and juicy as Prime cuts.

Preparing Leaner Meats

Preparing your meats with less fat can be simple and does not have to compromise taste. With a few simple tips, you can make a big difference in reducing total fat, saturated fat, and cholesterol in your meals. Try the following techniques:

- Trim all visible fat from meat before cooking.
- Cook meats using the following low-fat cooking methods most of the time: broil, grill, roast, braise, stew, steam, poach, stir-fry, or microwave.
- After browning ground meats, drain fat and then rinse meat in hot water a few times to rinse off excess fat. You can also pat the meat with a paper towel after draining to remove excess fat.
- Brown meat in a nonstick skillet with little to no fat. Use a vegetable oil spray to prevent sticking.
- When grilling, broiling, or roasting meat and poultry, use a rack for the fat to drip through.
- Use marinades for meat that have little to no fat such as light teriyaki sauce, orange juice, lime juice, lemon juice, tomato juice, defatted broth, or low-fat yogurt. Add fresh herbs and other spices such as garlic powder to marinades for more flavor.
- Oven bake fish and/or chicken instead of frying.

Keeping Meat Safe

The way you prepare, serve, and store meat can all add to its safety. Taking the proper care can ensure your meat will be high in quality and safe to eat. Take the following steps with your meats:

- Rinse poultry in cold water before preparing.
- Keep juices from meats and poultry from contacting other foods.
- Marinate meat and poultry in the refrigerator.
- Never reuse marinade once it is in contact with raw meat.
- Thaw frozen meat in the refrigerator or microwave.
- Use different utensils and cutting boards for raw meats than for cooked meats as well as other foods.
- Cook ground meat and poultry thoroughly. Use a meat thermometer

to ensure the internal temperature reaches around 160 degrees. The meat should no longer be pink inside, and juices should run clear.

- Cook other cuts of beef to at least 145 degrees for safety.
- Heat leftovers to 165 degrees or until steaming hot.
- Refrigerate leftovers promptly.

Milk, Yogurt, and Cheese Group

The milk or dairy group is also on the third level from the bottom of the Food Guide Pyramid, next to the meat group. The milk group includes milk and foods made from milk, such as yogurt, cheese, cottage cheese, buttermilk, frozen yogurt, and ice cream. The milk group, especially milk, yogurt, and cheese, is an excellent source of calcium and riboflavin. These foods provide many essential vitamins and minerals as well as protein. According to the National Dairy Council, "Intake of fluid milk has been demonstrated to reduce the risk of osteoporosis, hypertension, and colon cancer. Drinking milk may help to reduce the risk of kidney stones. Milk intake may help to reduce the risk of tooth decay by acting as a substitute for saliva."

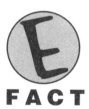

FACT

Even though some varieties of orange juice contain calcium, they should still be counted as a fruit and not as a dairy serving. Calcium is only one nutrient, and the nutrient content of juice is closer to a fruit than a dairy serving.

Fewer servings are needed from the milk group compared to other food groups because dairy foods are naturally higher in fat. Smaller amounts from the milk group will still provide the nutrients that you need. The Food Guide Pyramid suggests consuming two to three servings from the milk group each day.

One serving equals any of the following:

- 1 cup low-fat or fat-free milk
- 1 cup low-fat yogurt
- 1^1/2 ounces natural cheese
- 2 ounces processed cheese
- ^{1}/3 cup dry milk
- ^{3}/4 cup low-fat cottage cheese

Dairy foods are good sources of protein, calcium, riboflavin, phosphorus, potassium, vitamin A, and vitamin D. The dairy group is one of the biggest contributors to calcium intake, which is extremely important for bone health. Dairy foods are also a source of fat and cholesterol. Since dairy products are animal products, the majority of the fat they contain is saturated (the bad fat). Choosing lower-fat and fat-free versions can decrease fat and cholesterol intake. Skim milk has all the important nutrients in the same quantity as low-fat or whole milk. The only difference is the fat and calorie content.

Looking at Lactose

Dairy foods contain a natural occurring sugar called lactose. During digestion of dairy foods, an enzyme called lactase breaks down lactose to make it easily digestible. People who are lactose intolerant produce too little of this enzyme. Left undigested, lactose can cause nausea, cramping, bloating, gas, and diarrhea. Some people are more tolerant than others and can eat dairy products in different amounts. If you are lactose intolerant, choose low-lactose or lactose-free dairy products. A majority of lactose-intolerant people can eat yogurt with no symptoms.

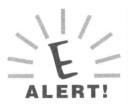

Lactose intolerance is *not* the same as a milk allergy. People who have a milk allergy are actually allergic to the protein in milk. People with milk allergies must avoid all milk products and any foods made from milk.

Safety Tips

As with any food group, it is important to choose your dairy products carefully and handle them properly for safety.

Tips for using dairy products safely include the following:

- Check the "sell-by" or "use-by" date on dairy products before purchasing. Examine containers for leaks and other damage.
- Buy only dairy foods that are properly refrigerated in the store.

- Keep dairy products properly chilled in your refrigerator at home. Temperatures above 40 degrees reduce the shelf life of milk and other milk products.
- Keep milk containers closed to prevent the absorption of other food flavors in the refrigerator.
- Never return unused milk to the original container.

Fats, Oils, and Sweets

Fats, oils, and sweets are concentrated at the tip of the Food Guide Pyramid. These foods include foods that are mostly fat or sugar, such as oils, salad dressings, cream, butter, gravy, margarine, cream cheese, soft drinks, candy, jams, gelatins, and fruit drinks. These foods supply calories but little in the way of nutrients. The tip of the pyramid is not considered a food group and has no recommended serving ranges because there are no minimum requirements for these foods. For most of the foods in the fat category, it is best to choose lower-fat versions such as low-fat cream cheese, sour cream, salad dressing, and the like. These foods add flavor to foods and can be part of a healthy diet if consumed in moderation. Enjoy foods that contain added sugars, such as soft drinks and candy, in moderation.

Putting the Pyramid Together

The idea behind the Food Guide Pyramid is not to try to design each one of your meals after it but to use it as a daily or weekly guide. The key is to eat, on average, according to the guidelines in the pyramid. If your present diet does not meet the recommendations, begin to make small changes until you can, on average, eat the way the pyramid instructs. Make small changes one at a time such as adding a fruit at breakfast, adding a vegetable at lunch, or switching to skim milk or low-fat salad dressing. Gradual changes are more apt to become a permanent part of your lifestyle than radical ones. (E)

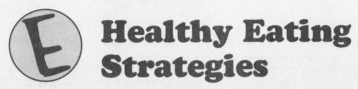

Chapter 4

Healthy Eating Strategies

Adopting healthier eating habits does not have to be difficult, and it can put you quickly on your way to improved health. With a little bit of effort you can make changes in your eating patterns that can make a substantial difference in your health. The key is being willing to change habits and adopt new ones.

Get a Head Start with Breakfast

Breakfast is one of the most important meals, yet it is probably the most skipped meal of the day. The word "breakfast" describes exactly what it does: breaks a fast. After a good night's rest, your body has gone eight to twelve hours without food or energy. It needs to replenish its blood sugar stores. Blood sugar, or glucose, which comes from the breakdown of food in the body, is your body's main source of energy. Eating food provides your body with a fresh supply of blood glucose or energy. The brain in particular needs a fresh supply of glucose each day because that is its main source of energy. (The brain does not store glucose.) Eating breakfast is associated with being more productive and efficient in the morning hours. Breakfast eaters tend to experience better concentration, problem-solving ability, strength, and endurance. Your muscles also rely on a fresh supply of blood glucose for physical activity throughout the day.

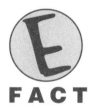

FACT

According to the United States Department of Agriculture (USDA), breakfast should provide 18 percent of Americans' daily intake of calories and 12 to 28 percent of their daily intake of vitamins and minerals. Studies have shown that people who skip breakfast tend to be heavier than those who make time to eat a nutritious breakfast.

Don't have time for breakfast? Get up a few minutes earlier. You don't need a lot of time to prepare a nutritious breakfast. Just a small amount of healthful food can help refuel your body properly and will be worth the few minutes of lost sleep. Keep quick breakfast foods on hand, or get your breakfast foods ready the night before to save time in the morning. Avoid fast foods. While it's tempting to stop at the drive-through, these meals aren't going to do much for you in terms of health and nutrition.

Do you think that eating breakfast might make you gain weight? Eating a good healthy breakfast can help regulate your appetite throughout the day. Breakfast can help you eat in moderation at lunch and dinner. Also, research indicates that a high-fiber, low-fat breakfast may make a major contribution to a total reduced fat intake for the day.

If you have a hard time facing food first thing in the morning, start with eating a light breakfast, such as a piece of toast or fruit. Pack a breakfast or snack to take with you so you can eat once you do get hungry.

Eating a nutritious breakfast gets you off to a healthy start each morning. You will feel and perform your best. If you are not a breakfast eater, start slow and introduce at least one food every morning, such as a glass of juice or a low-fat yogurt. Then work your way up to a little bit more of a substantial breakfast. Here are some quick breakfast meals to help you get started:

- Cold cereal with fruit and skim milk
- Yogurt with fruit or low-fat granola cereal
- Peanut butter on a whole-wheat bagel and orange juice
- Bran muffin and a banana
- Instant oatmeal with raisins or berries
- Breakfast smoothie (blend fruit and skim milk)
- Hard-boiled egg and grapefruit juice
- Cottage cheese and peaches

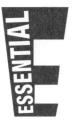

It *does* matter what foods you eat at breakfast. Eating high-sugar foods, such as doughnuts or sugary cereals, will cause a quick rise in your blood sugar, resulting in a temporary energy surge. After about an hour, your blood sugar will decline and bring on symptoms of hunger. When you eat a well-balanced breakfast, your body gets a sustained release of energy and delays symptoms of hunger for several hours by maintaining your blood sugar levels.

Don't Skip Meals

You need to fuel your body throughout the day with nutritious foods for optimal energy and performance. Skipping meals can have numerous negative effects on your healthy lifestyle. Skipping meals can make you so hungry that you overeat at your next eating opportunity. Not only will you probably overeat at the next meal, but chances are you won't eat as healthily either. Skipping meals can affect your productivity, concentration, and energy level throughout the day. Finally, skipping meals increases the chance that you will not consume all of your needed servings from the Food Guide Pyramid. So make time and even schedule eating opportunities throughout the day.

Not having time does not mean you have to give up on eating a healthy diet. Your time is precious, so try some of these tips to help you save time yet not miss meals:

- When you do have time to cook, make double and triple batches and store them in the freezer. For example, if you are making spaghetti, make an extra batch of sauce and freeze it.
- If you have days off during the week or are free on weekends, do some of your prep work for the week and freeze it. Cook and cut up chicken for a casserole and store it in individual meal containers for quick thawing during the week.
- Stock your kitchen with quick-fix foods such as frozen vegetables, lean burgers, salsa (great mixed with rice or to top chicken breasts), salad ingredients, pasta, and rice.
- Use quick cooking methods such as grilling, microwaving, or stir-frying.
- Use a slow cooker. Put your meal in before you leave for work, and come home to a hot cooked meal.
- Prepare meals that pack a variety of food groups into one dish, such as casseroles or one-pan dishes.
- Buy prepared foods to help you save time, such as precut stir-fry vegetables, low-fat grated cheese, skinless chicken strips, washed spinach, and frozen chopped onions.

Slow Down!

Slow down, enjoy, and actually taste your food. It takes at least twenty minutes for your stomach to signal your brain that it is full. Slowing down will help to curb the urge to go back for a second helping. Slowing down can also help to ensure proper digestion. To help yourself slow down, take sips of your beverage between bites, put your fork down in between bites, and enjoy the conversation of others. Sit down to eat instead of eating while standing at the counter, driving, or watching television. Eating while doing other things means you are eating unconsciously, and you may consume more than you plan to.

Controlling Portion Sizes

Portion sizes are crucial when you're trying to eat a healthy diet. In fact, one of the primary reasons people are overweight is lack of portion control. To follow the Food Guide Pyramid guidelines, you need to be aware of serving or portion sizes. Serving sizes are specific, standardized amounts of food and are meant as general guidelines to help you plan and judge your own portions. The portion sizes you consume contribute directly to the amount of calories and the amount of fat that you consume per day.

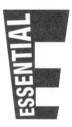

The best approach to ensuring that you don't skip meals is to plan your meals and snacks ahead of time. Planning ahead is the key to eating a healthy diet throughout the day. This will also help to prevent haphazard eating, which often results in high-calorie, high-fat eating.

To follow a healthy diet, you don't need to weigh and measure all of your food each day. Keep in mind that portion sizes are meant as general guidelines, so the aim is to come close to the recommended serving sizes, on average, over several days. Use these visual comparisons to help estimate your portion sizes:

- A 3-ounce portion of cooked meat, poultry, or fish is about the size of a deck of playing cards.
- A medium potato is about the size of a computer mouse.
- 1 cup of rice or pasta is about the size of a fist or a tennis ball.
- An average bagel should be the size of a hockey puck or a large to-go coffee lid.

- A cup of fruit or a medium apple or orange is the size of a baseball.
- ½ cup of chopped vegetables is about the size of three regular ice cubes.
- 3 ounces of grilled fish is the size of your checkbook.
- 1 ounce of cheese is the size of four dice.
- 1 teaspoon of peanut butter equals one die; 2 tablespoons is about the size of a golf ball.
- 1 ounce of snack foods—pretzels, etc.—equals a large handful.
- 1 thumb tip equals 1 teaspoon; 3 thumb tips equal 1 tablespoon; and a whole thumb equals 1 ounce.

To help you eat only the portions you measure out, portion out your food before bringing it to the table. You will be less likely to eat more when serving bowls are not on the table. Another clever trick is to use a smaller plate to make your portion sizes look bigger.

Smart Snacking

Contrary to popular belief, snacking can be part of a healthful eating plan. Choosing snacks wisely can help fuel your body between meals, give you an energy boost, and add to your total intake of essential nutrients for the day. Snacking can also help to take the edge off hunger between meals. The longer you wait between meals, the more you tend to eat at the next meal. Leaving only about three to four hours between meals is an ideal amount of time to keep blood sugar levels in control. The key to smart snacking is the type and amounts of food that you choose. Mindless snacking or nibbling on high-fat, high-calorie foods can lead to trouble in the form of unwanted and empty calories.

To make snacking a healthy part of your diet, try these tips:

- Choose snacks that are lower in fat and nutrient rich.
- Make snacks part of your eating plan for the day instead of thinking of them as an extra.
- Make snacking a conscious activity.

- Plan and eat snacks well ahead of mealtime.
- Eat smaller portion snacks, not meal-size ones.

Try some of these smart snacks as part of your healthy eating plan:

- ½ bagel with peanut butter
- Raw vegetables with low-fat or fat-free dressing
- Fruit yogurt topped with low-fat granola cereal
- Low-fat cottage cheese topped with fresh fruit
- Fresh fruit
- Light microwave popcorn
- Pita bread stuffed with fresh veggies and low-fat dressing
- Low-fat string cheese
- Whole-grain cereal and fat-free milk
- Vegetable juice

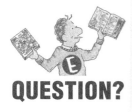

QUESTION?

Can eating smaller meals more than three times a day be part of a healthy diet?
Yes. Eating small meals means eating smaller portion meals throughout the day, with the same goals of variety, balance, and moderation. For healthful grazing make sure you still get your needed number of servings from all of the food groups. Balance the amount of food you eat, and eat smaller portions.

Curious about Caffeine?

Caffeine is a substance that occurs naturally in certain plants, including coffee, tea, cocoa beans, and kola nuts. Many people drink coffee or caffeinated products to get themselves going or to prevent fatigue. People ingest caffeine mostly from colas, soft drinks, coffee, tea, chocolate, caffeinated water, over-the-counter drugs, and prescription drugs. There are more than a thousand different over-the-counter and prescription drugs that list caffeine as an ingredient. There is even a very small amount of caffeine in decaffeinated coffee.

Caffeine can be safe and can be part of a healthy eating plan if consumed in moderation and not used to take the place of healthier fluids such as water, fruit juice, and milk. There is currently no scientific evidence that links moderate amounts of caffeine to any health risk such as cancer, heart disease, birth defects, or fibrocystic breast disease.

Effects of Caffeine

Caffeine is considered a mild stimulant. Caffeine affects the central nervous system by temporarily increasing heart rate and blood pressure. For some people this can cause effects such as jitters and anxiety. Caffeine can irritate the stomach, cause headaches, and can even cause insomnia. Caffeine can also slightly increase the amount of calcium lost from the body. Caffeine can have a diuretic effect by increasing water lost through urination. The more caffeine you consume, the greater its potential to increase water loss. Because of caffeine's diuretic effects, caffeine-containing beverages are not the best choice of fluids. The effects of caffeine don't last long since caffeine is not stored in the body. Within three to four hours, most of the caffeine is excreted, and the effects decrease.

How Much Is Too Much?

The question of how much caffeine is too much depends on your individual tolerance. You may want to think about cutting back on your caffeine intake if you are consuming caffeinated beverages in place of juice or milk or if your intake is more than 200 to 300 milligrams a day (about 2 cups of coffee). For most healthy adults, consuming 200 to 300 milligrams a day poses no physical problems.

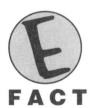

An average 12-ounce cola contains about 35 milligrams of caffeine, while an average 8-ounce cup of brewed coffee contains about 85 milligrams of caffeine. Keep in mind, too, that soft drinks other than colas also contain caffeine, sometimes even more.

Some people are more sensitive to caffeine and may feel the effects more easily. Others can develop a tolerance to caffeine over time and not notice the effects as quickly. If you have questions about caffeine and your health, you should consult your personal physician.

Who Should Cut Back?

In moderation, you can enjoy caffeine-containing beverages as part of your healthy lifestyle. People who may want to think about cutting back include pregnant or breastfeeding women; people with certain medical problems, such as high blood pressure or ulcers; younger children; and older adults. Sensitivity can increase during pregnancy, and caffeine can be passed to the baby through breast milk. Older adults may also experience an increased sensitivity to the effects of caffeine. Children, because of their smaller size, can easily drink enough caffeine to cause restlessness, anxiety, and jitters. At any age you should watch how much caffeine you consume each day.

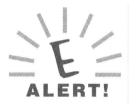

ALERT!

If you struggle with insomnia, you should avoid caffeine in the evening hours. Caffeine only takes fifteen to twenty minutes to get into your blood, and the caffeine effect lasts for about three to four hours. Keep in mind to read medication labels carefully if you are trying to decrease or avoid caffeine intake. Over-the-counter pain relief tablets often contain as much caffeine as 1 or 2 cups of coffee.

To cut back, it is best to reduce caffeine intake slowly, especially if you have been ingesting heavy amounts of caffeine for some time. A gradual cutback can help you to avoid the temporary headache, restlessness, and drowsiness that can occur. If you currently drink more than 3 cups of coffee per day, cut down by a cup every three or four days until you are down to 3 cups. This will help reduce the symptoms of caffeine withdrawal. Try mixing half decaf and half regular coffee or drinking instant instead of brewed coffee; instant coffee is lower in caffeine than brewed coffee. Or replace your afternoon soda with a glass of juice or a glass of water—you'll get more nutrients without the caffeine.

Caffeine and Anxiety

According to the National Coffee Association, 80 percent of Americans drink coffee, and occasional coffee consumption rose 6 percent in the last year. At the same time, panic and other anxiety disorders have become the most common mental illnesses in the United States. Professionals agree that when caffeine overlaps with these disorders, the result can be trouble. Psychologist Norman B. Schmidt, Ph.D., states, "If you tend to be a high-strung, anxious person, using a lot of caffeine can be risky." Roland Griffiths, Ph.D., a professor in the Departments of Psychiatry and Neuroscience at the John Hopkins University School of Medicine states, "Caffeine is the most widely used mood-altering drug in the world. People often see coffee, tea, and soft drinks simply as beverages rather than vehicles for a psychoactive drug. But caffeine can exacerbate anxiety and panic disorders."

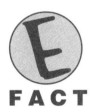

FACT

If you experience problems with anxiety, panic attacks, or nervousness, try to drastically, but slowly, cut down or cut caffeine out of your diet altogether. Cutting caffeine from your diet will not cure your anxiety problems but may help decrease symptoms.

Hunger vs. Cravings

The question is, is it a craving, or am I really hungry? We first need to understand the difference between a physical food craving—or actual hunger—and an emotional food craving. Cravings can be caused by either physical or psychological needs. Emotional cravings or eating triggers are usually caused by psychological needs, while hunger is a biological function of the body's real need for food. Emotional cravings can lead to bingeing. Learn to listen to your body, and know what it is trying to tell you.

The key is trusting yourself to know whether you are craving a food for emotional reasons or whether your body is truly hungry. Giving in to too many cravings can lead to overeating, unhealthy eating, and extra weight gain. Healthy eating means eating when you are truly hungry and eating until you are satisfied. It is being able to choose healthy foods but not being so restrictive that you miss out on foods you really enjoy.

You can use many techniques to distinguish between biological and emotional cravings. Use these descriptions to classify a physical craving versus an emotional craving.

A physical craving has the following qualities:

- You are physiologically hungry.
- The craving does not go away if you try to wait it out.
- The craving intensifies over time.
- Nothing you do will take away the craving except the craved food.

An emotional craving, on the other hand, looks like this:

- You are not physiologically hungry.
- It does go away if you try to wait it out.
- The craving does not intensify over time; the emotion does.
- Doing something else satisfies the real need, and the craving disappears.

Hunger Signals

Being aware of your body's physical hunger signals helps give you the confidence to satisfy your food cravings. Hunger signals can come from your stomach while it is informing you that it is empty or from your brain as it informs you that it is lacking an energy supply. Signals from your stomach may include growls, pangs, or hollow feelings. Signals from your brain may include fogginess, lack of concentration, headache, or fatigue. If you still are not sure whether you are truly hungry, try using the following Hunger/Fullness Rating Scale.

10	Absolutely, positively stuffed
9	So full that it hurts
8	Very full and bloated
7	Starting to feel uncomfortable
6	Slightly overeaten
5	Perfectly comfortable
4	First signals that your body needs food
3	Strong signals to eat
2	Very hungry, irritable
1	Extreme hunger, dizziness

If you are at level 5 or above, you are not hungry and your body does not physically need food. If you are craving a food, it is emotional, not physical. If you are at level 3 or 4, your body is telling you that it needs some food, and your cravings are telling you that you physically need food. If you are at level 1 or 2, your body is too hungry and definitely physically needs food. The problem on waiting until you get to this level is that you are so hungry that you will probably overeat or eat something that is not as healthy.

The best time to eat is at level 3 or 4. At this point you are experiencing physical hunger, and your body is telling you that you need food. You still have enough control to eat healthful foods and control your portion sizes.

Craving Solutions

When you are craving foods, it is important to determine whether the craving is physical or emotional. Once you have discovered why you want to eat, you can take action. If you determine it is emotional, take steps to try to dissolve your craving in some other way than giving in to the food. For instance, bingeing or emotional cravings can happen due to stress. Stress reduction techniques might include taking a long hot bath, taking a walk, relaxation exercises, or yoga. Drink a glass of water before giving in to a craving. Sometimes when you think you're hungry, you're really just thirsty. If you are not only truly hungry but overly hungry, eat something healthy, such as carrot sticks or an apple, instead of junk food you may be craving. That may fill you up enough to disband unhealthy food cravings. Use the ten-minute rule. When you crave something, wait for ten minutes for the craving to subside. Another option is to satisfy your craving with a very small portion of what you are craving.

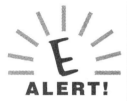

ALERT!

Never consume fewer than 1,200 calories when trying to lose weight. Below 1,200 calories, your body cannot obtain the proper amount of nutrients required for optimal health. Also, lowering your calories too much can slow down your metabolism, or the rate at which your body burns calories, making it harder to lose and easier to gain the weight back.

Studies suggest that completely avoiding certain foods can make them irresistible and make you crave them even more. The result is that you usually will give in to the craving, overindulge, and then feel guilty for letting it happen. If you are truly physically hungry, eat (in moderation, of course). Keep in mind that you are hungrier on some days than others. So when you're really, truly hungry, it's fine to eat more. Remember that one meal does not define healthy eating habits. What you eat over the course of a day, or actually over several days, does. Healthy eating is flexible. Giving in to a craving, in moderation, can be part of a healthy eating pattern as long as it does not get out of hand.

Eating Triggers

Many things can trigger our desire to eat. The aroma of food, the sight of a favorite food, a commercial on television, or just knowing that there are sweets in the house. The habit of eating while watching television can make television an eating trigger. Recognizing what triggers eating or cravings is the first step in learning to control them.

Keeping a food diary can help identify your eating triggers. This can help you notice when you eat and what you are doing or thinking when you have a craving. If you find that sitting in front of the television is a major trigger for cravings, plan to do something when you are in that situation. Take up knitting, write letters, or pay your bills when you are watching television. Do something that will keep your hands busy and keep your mind off the desire to eat. If boredom is a trigger, make a list of alternate activities, such as talking to a friend, taking a walk, or washing the car. When you get bored and want to eat, check out your list instead.

The key to cravings and triggers is to learn to recognize them and then to set up an action plan to help you deal with them. Cravings are a very normal part of our lives, and it is important to a healthy eating plan to deal with them in a sensible manner.

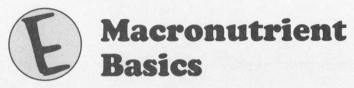

Chapter 5

Macronutrient Basics

Nutrients are grouped into six different categories: carbohydrates, proteins, fats, vitamins, minerals, and water. Carbohydrates, proteins, and fats are called "macronutrients" because we need larger amounts in our diet. Some foods consist of one, two, or all three of these macronutrients. It is important for your body to acquire all three for proper functioning.

Macronutrient Needs

Even though each macronutrient has a particular function in the body, they work in partnership for good health. Our bodies need all three macronutrients to function properly, but not in equal amounts. Some evidence suggests that a poor energy mix in the diet is a risk factor for diseases like coronary heart disease and certain cancers.

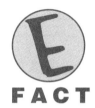

FACT

Keep in mind that there are 4 calories per gram of carbohydrate and protein and 9 calories per gram of fat.

Most health professionals recommend that we eat a daily diet made up of approximately 55 percent carbohydrates, 15 percent protein, and no more than 30 percent total fat. Following the Food Guide Pyramid will ensure you are consuming optimal amounts of each macronutrient. If you want to get more specific, you can easily figure out how many calories and grams of each macronutrient you need for good health by using the following equations.

Figure Your Carbohydrate Need

Multiply your calorie intake by .55 to determine how many calories you should get from carbohydrates. Divide that number by 4 calories/gram to find the total number of carbohydrates (in grams) that you should eat. (For example: 1,600 calories multiplied by .55 equals 880 calories from carbohydrates; 880 calories from carbohydrates divided by 4 calories/gram equals 220 grams of carbohydrates.)

Figure Your Protein Need

Multiply your calorie intake by .15 to find how many calories you should get from protein. Divide that by 4 calories/gram to find the amount (in grams) of protein you should eat. (For example: 1,600 calories multiplied by .15 equals 240 calories from protein; 240 calories from protein divided by 4 calories/gram equals 60 grams of protein.)

Figure Your Fat Need

Multiply your calorie intake by .30 to find how many calories you need from fat. Then divide that by 9 calories/gram for the total amount of fat (in grams) you should eat. (For example: 1,600 calories multiplied by .30 equals 480 calories from fat; 480 calories from fat divided by 9 calories/gram equals 53 grams of fat.)

Crazy for Carbohydrates

Carbohydrates are your body's main source of energy, especially for the brain and nervous system. A nutrient that provides energy also provides calories. Carbohydrates are made up of carbon, hydrogen, and oxygen molecules. Carbohydrates are found in fruits, vegetables, dairy products, starches, and foods in the meat group such as beans and soy products. The only food they are not found in is meat.

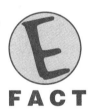

FACT

Legumes come from plants and are part of the dried bean, pea, and lentil family. They include beans of types such as black, garbanzo, lima, navy, soy, kidney, and pinto, as well as lentils. Legumes are rich in fiber, protein, complex carbohydrates, B vitamins, and other vitamins and minerals. Legumes are part of the meat group, but they also fit into the vegetable group in the Food Guide Pyramid because they provide complex carbohydrates as well as protein.

Carbohydrates are classified into two different categories: simple carbohydrates (sugars) and complex carbohydrates (starches). Sugars are carbohydrates in their simplest form. Refined sugars are found in foods such as table sugar, honey, jams, candy, syrup, and soft drinks. Refined sugars provide calories, but they lack vitamins, minerals, and fiber. Some simple sugars, such as naturally occurring sugars, are found in more nutritious foods. These include sugars such as fructose found in fruit and lactose found in dairy products. Complex carbohydrates are basically many simple sugars linked together. Complex carbohydrates are found in foods such as grains, pasta, rice, vegetables, breads, legumes, nuts, and seeds.

Fiber is also considered a carbohydrate and is important to health. However, fiber is not considered a nutrient, because most of it is not digested or absorbed into the body.

How Much?

Healthy adults should consume approximately 55 percent of their total daily calories from carbohydrates. That means filling more than half of your plate with carbohydrate-rich foods such as grains, fruits, vegetables, and beans. The idea is to eat larger amounts of carbohydrates and smaller portions of protein and fat.

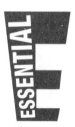

It is estimated that American adults get almost 20 percent of their daily total calories from sugar. On a 2,000-calorie diet, that is 400 calories, equivalent to 25 teaspoons of sugar a day! The ideal intake of sugar is no more than 10 percent of total calories, about 200 calories on a 2,000-calorie diet.

Ounce for ounce, starches contain the same number of calories as protein and less than half the calories of fat. Carbohydrates and protein provide 4 calories per gram, and fat provides 9 calories per gram. Complex carbohydrates such as grains, vegetables, and legumes should supply the bulk of your carbohydrate calories since they supply a good bonus of vitamins, minerals, and fiber. Some simple carbohydrates, mostly refined and processed sugars, are sometimes referred to as "empty calories" or calories that provide energy (calories) but no nutritional value. In addition, high-sugar foods mix with the bacteria in plaque and increase your risk for tooth decay.

To increase complex carbohydrates, use the following tips:

- Eat more fruits and vegetables.
- Eat more whole grains, rice, breads, and cereals.
- Eat more beans, lentils, and dried peas.

How They Work

All carbohydrates, whether simple or complex, must first be converted into glucose to be used as fuel or energy for the body. Because glucose circulates in your bloodstream, it is also known as blood sugar. From your bloodstream, glucose enters your body's cells, where it is converted to energy. Since simple carbohydrates, or simple sugars, are already in their simplest form, they go straight into the bloodstream. Complex carbohydrates must first be broken down by digestive enzymes into glucose.

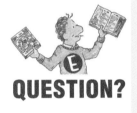

QUESTION?

Is it true that eating carbohydrates can make you fat?
No. Carbohydrates alone will not make you fat. Eating too many calories—from carbohydrates, proteins, or fat—or going overboard on any type of food or nutrient will cause weight gain. A deficiency of carbohydrates in your diet can cause a lack of calories (malnutrition) or excessive intake of fat to make up the lost calories.

The body does not turn all its blood sugar or glucose into energy at the same time. Some glucose is used immediately for energy and some is stored for future use. Glucose is stored in the liver and muscles in the form of glycogen. If you consume more calories than you need, excess glucose is also stored as fat. After you eat, the hormone insulin lowers the level of glucose in the blood by stimulating body cells to take up and store excess glucose. This helps to prevent your blood sugar from spiking too high. Another job of insulin is to help prevent too much glucose in the liver from being released between meals. At times when your blood sugar is low, such as after exercising or before breakfast, another hormone called glucagon stimulates the conversion of glycogen from the liver back to glucose for the body to use as energy. In simpler terms, insulin helps to regulate your blood sugar.

Protein Power

Protein is another macronutrient that is important to a healthy diet. Like carbohydrates, protein is made up of carbon, hydrogen, and oxygen. But proteins also contain nitrogen, which makes their role in the body's health unique. The body uses protein to build and repair bone, muscles, connective tissue, skin, internal organs, and blood. Protein also makes up your hair, nails, and teeth. Hormones, antibodies, and enzymes, which regulate the body's chemical reactions, are all composed of protein. Protein helps wounds to heal and blood to clot. If carbohydrates and fats can't meet your body's energy needs, protein can also be used as an energy source, because it provides calories.

Protein can be found in meat, poultry, fish, eggs, milk, cheese, yogurt, and soy products. Legumes, seeds, and nuts also supply protein. Grain products and some vegetables supply smaller amounts of protein. Since animal products do provide the majority of protein in the typical American diet, and animal products contain saturated fat and cholesterol, it is important to choose lower-fat dairy products and lean cuts of meat.

Amino Acids

Protein is made up of building blocks called amino acids. There are about twenty different amino acids in the body. These amino acids are linked in thousands of different ways to form thousands of different types of proteins. Each of these proteins has a unique function in the body. The amino acids must be arranged in a precise way to carry out their proper function. Deoxyribonucleic acid, or DNA, is the genetic code that carries instructions for the arrangement of each protein.

Nine amino acids are classified as essential because your body does not make them and must get them from the foods you eat. Other amino acids are classified as nonessential because your body will make them if you consume enough essential amino acids and enough calories.

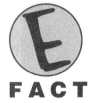

FACT

Soy is the only plant food that contains all nine essential amino acids in sufficient proportions to be considered a complete protein.

Your body cannot directly use the protein you consume. Digestive enzymes break protein down into short amino-acid chains and then finally into individual amino acids. These amino acids can then enter the bloodstream and travel to the cells, where the body rebuilds them into the sequence or into the type of protein that it needs for a specific task. The body continually gets the amino acids it needs from a diet that meets your protein needs and from its own amino-acid pool.

In general, animal proteins contain all nine of the essential amino acids and are therefore considered complete proteins. Foods such as legumes, vegetables, grains, nuts, and seeds are considered incomplete proteins because they are missing sufficient quantities of one or more essential amino acids.

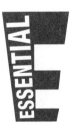

ESSENTIAL

If you do not eat animal foods, there is no need to combine specific foods at each meal to get all of your essential amino acids. If you eat enough calories and eat a variety of plant foods, your body will get enough amino acids to make its own complete proteins.

How Much?

Protein needs are specific to your age and gender. **TABLE 5-1** gives the Recommended Daily Allowances (RDA) of protein for a variety of categories.

Table 5-1 Recommended Daily Protein		
Category	**Age or Condition**	**Protein Grams**
Infants	Up to 5 months	13 grams
	5 months to 1 year	14 grams
Children	1 to 3 years	16 grams
	4 to 6 years	24 grams
	7 to 10 years	28 grams
Males	11 to 14 years	45 grams
	15 to 18 years	59 grams
	19 to 24 years	58 grams
	25 to 50 years	63 grams
	51-plus years	63 grams
Females	11 to 14 years	46 grams
	15 to 18 years	44 grams
	19 to 24 years	46 grams
	25 to 50 years	50 grams
	51-plus years	50 grams
Pregnant		60 grams
Breastfeeding	First 6 months	65 grams
	Second 6 months	62 grams

It is not hard to get your needed protein for the day. The numbers can add up quickly. Keep in mind the following protein contents of common foods:

- A 3- to 4-ounce serving of lean meat, poultry, or fish contains about 25 to 35 grams of protein per day. That is approximately the size of a deck of cards.
- 1 cup of cooked beans or lentils contains about 18 grams of protein.
- 1 cup of low-fat or fat-free milk contains 8 grams of protein.

- 1 cup of low-fat yogurt contains about 10 grams of protein.
- 1 cup of low-fat cottage cheese contains about 28 grams of protein.
- 2 tablespoons of peanut butter contains about 7 grams of protein.
- 2 ounces of low-fat cheese contains about 14 to 16 grams of protein.
- 1 egg contains about 7 grams of protein.
- 1 serving of vegetables contains around 1 to 3 grams of protein.
- 1 serving of grain foods generally contains 3 to 6 grams of protein.

Athletes and Protein Intake

Whether you are an athlete, an avid exerciser, or neither, you need protein in your diet. Protein is needed for the development of muscle, but you do not need more protein to build bigger muscles. The only thing that builds bigger muscles is exercise and working your muscles. Consuming extra amounts of protein from either food or supplements really has no added benefit. Athletes only need slightly more protein than the RDAs. Generally non-athletes need around ½ gram per pound of body weight and most athletes need ½ to ¾ grams of protein per pound of body weight.

Too Much Protein

When you consume too much protein, either from food or from supplements, the body uses only what it needs. Extra protein is not stored in the body as protein for future use. Excess protein is either used as energy or stored as body fat.

Eating large amounts of protein, especially from animal foods, can increase your saturated fat (bad fat) and cholesterol intake. It can also cause nutrient imbalances by crowding out other important foods such as grains, fruits, and vegetables.

Too much protein can actually be harmful to the body. It puts an extra strain on the kidneys. When protein is digested, it produces by-products that are toxic to the body, and it is the kidney's job to filter out these toxins. Excess protein makes the kidneys work harder. Dehydration can also be a problem. When you consume excess protein, you need more water to excrete the urea, a waste product formed when protein turns to body fat. This increases the chances for dehydration and increases the need to urinate.

The Skinny on Fat

Fat is another macronutrient vital to a healthy diet. With all the negative things you hear about fat today, it is important to remember that fat is a necessary nutrient in the diet. Like carbohydrates and proteins, fat provides energy, which means it provides calories. In fact, fat is a very concentrated source of energy, providing more than double the amount of calories in one gram of carbohydrate or protein. Fats are made up of carbon, hydrogen, and oxygen molecules. The general term for fat found in food is triglyceride.

We need moderate amounts of fat in our diets to perform important functions. Fat helps carry, absorb, and store the fat-soluble vitamins (A, D, E, and K) in your bloodstream. Without fat, these vitamins would not be able to nourish the body. Fat can also be used as an energy source. The body saves extra fat in your body's fat cells. When you need extra energy, your body can use these fat stores. A certain amount of body fat is needed to cushion your organs and protect them from injury and to supply insulation to help regulate body temperature.

How Much?

Health experts agree that you should get no more than 30 percent of your total calories from fat. They also recommend consuming no more than 10 percent of that 30 percent from saturated sources of fat and no more than 7 percent if you have coronary heart disease, diabetes, or high-LDL cholesterol. Eating any type of fat in excess can cause weight gain because it is higher in calories. Overloading on specific types of fat, such as saturated fat, can also put you at risk for serious health problems.

Sorting Out the Fats

Not only is it important to watch how much fat you eat, but it is also important to pay attention to the type of fat you eat. There are different types of triglycerides or dietary fat. Some of these fats are more harmful than others. The major kinds of fats in the foods we eat are saturated, polyunsaturated, monounsaturated, and trans fatty acids.

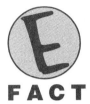

FACT

Cholesterol is not the same thing as fat. Cholesterol is a fatlike substance, but it has a different structure and different functions. Also, cholesterol does not provide energy to the body; therefore, it has no calories.

Saturated fatty acids have all the hydrogen the carbon atoms can hold on their chemical chains. Foods high in saturated fats are usually solid at room temperature. Saturated fats are one of the main dietary factors in raising blood cholesterol. A high blood-cholesterol level is a major risk factor for coronary heart disease, which can lead to a heart attack and can also increase the risk of stroke. The major sources of saturated fat are animal foods, such as meat, poultry, and whole-milk dairy products. A few plant sources contain saturated fat, including palm, palm kernel, and coconut oils.

Trans fatty acids are produced when unsaturated fats undergo a process called hydrogenation. Some trans fats are found naturally in foods, but most come from the hydrogenation of fat. Hydrogenation is a process that makes unsaturated fats—liquid and semisoft fat—stable and solid at room temperature. Trans fatty acids can be harmful because the body uses them much like saturated fats, and they are another main dietary factor in raising blood cholesterol. They raise LDL cholesterol (the bad cholesterol) and tend to lower HDL cholesterol (the good cholesterol). Margarine is an example of trans fats or hydrogenated fats. Tub margarine in its liquid form is unsaturated, but with the hydrogenation process it becomes semisoft. With even more hydrogenation, it becomes even harder and forms stick margarine. Other foods that contain trans fats include cookies, crackers, and other commercial baked goods made with partially hydrogenated vegetable oils as well as French fries, doughnuts, and other commercial fried foods. Reducing your total fat intake and limiting processed products that contain partially hydrogenated oils can significantly reduce your intake of trans fatty acids.

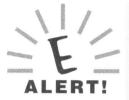

ALERT!

The American Heart Association states, "Hydrogenated fats in margarine and other fats are acceptable if the product contains liquid vegetable oil as the first ingredient and no more than 2 grams of saturated fat per tablespoon. The fatty-acid content of most margarines and spreads is printed on the label. Liquid and soft tub margarines contain little saturated fat or trans fat."

There are two types of unsaturated fats. The first is monounsaturated fats. Monounsaturated fats are liquid at room temperature but start to solidify at refrigerated temperatures. These fatty acids are missing one hydrogen pair on their chemical chain; in other words, they have one spot that is not saturated. Sources of monounsaturated fats include certain plant oils, such as olive, canola, and peanut oils. Avocados are also good sources of monounsaturated fats.

Polyunsaturated fats are liquid at room temperature as well as at refrigerated temperatures. These fatty acids are missing more than one hydrogen pair; that is, they have several spots on their chemical chain that are not saturated. Sources of polyunsaturated fats also include certain plant oils such as corn, cotton seed, safflower, sunflower, sesame, and soybean oils. Nuts and seeds are also good sources. The fat in fish is also a polyunsaturated fat.

There are two polyunsaturated essential fatty acids that your body does not make, and you must get these from the food you consume. These two fatty acids are linoleic acid (or omega-6) and linolenic acid (or omega-3). Children need these essential fatty acids to grow properly, and adults need them to maintain healthy skin and hair. Some new findings have reported that omega-3 fatty acids may have a beneficial effect on cardiovascular disease.

Both polyunsaturated and monounsaturated fats can help to lower blood cholesterol levels when they are consumed in larger quantities than saturated fats in the diet. Not only is it important to watch *what type* of fat you consume, it is important to watch *how much* fat you consume. All types of fat should be consumed in moderation because whether they are saturated or unsaturated, they contain twice as many calories as protein or carbohydrates.

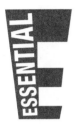

The American Heart Association recommends eating fish at least two times per week. Some fatty fish, such as mackerel, herring, lake trout, sardines, albacore tuna, and salmon, are high in omega-3 fatty acids, which may provide important health benefits.

Low-Fat Living

It is important to include fat in your daily diet but in moderation. Eating a completely fat-free diet is *not* part of a healthy eating style. To help you incorporate fat in moderation in your diet, use some of the following tips:

- Choose low-fat or fat-free dairy products such as skim milk; 1-percent milk; low-fat cheese, sour cream, and yogurt; and reduced-fat ice creams.
- Buy low-fat dressings and use those that are higher in saturated fats, such as buttermilk ranch or blue cheese, less often.
- Use nonstick cooking sprays or nonstick pans instead of frying with large amounts of oil or butter.
- Trim excess fat and skin from poultry.
- Look at food labels for amount of total fat and type of fat.
- Watch for hidden fats in your foods, such as toppings on pizza, fried foods, ice cream, high-fat meats (salami, bologna, bratwurst, hot dogs, pepperoni, sausage, bacon, and spare ribs), cakes, cookies, macaroni salad, potato salad, and coleslaw.
- Limit your intake of red meat, especially higher-fat cuts. Opt for poultry, fish, or nonmeat dishes more often.
- Watch for ingredient lists and fat content on margarines.
- Substitute lower-fat toppings for butter or margarine on foods such as

vegetables and potatoes. Try using salsa, low-fat, or fat-free salad dressings, herbs, and/or spices.

• Watch out for pastas in cream sauces. Use marinara or other tomato-based toppings instead.

Dietary Supplements

Eating a healthy and varied diet can provide the ideal mixture of vitamins, minerals, and other nutrients. However, even people with the best intentions sometimes fall short of their nutritional needs.

Today the definition of dietary supplements covers vitamins, minerals, fiber, herbs, other botanicals, amino acids, concentrates, and extracts. Ideally it is best to get all of your necessary nutrients from your diet and not from popping a pill. The body more readily absorbs nutrients when they come from the foods we eat. Although pill popping is not the recommended way to get the vitamins and minerals you need, some people do need assistance to receive their required daily allowances.

Who Should Take Supplements

There are some people who may benefit from taking supplements. Look at your diet and ask yourself whether you do these things on most days:

• Eat 6 to 11 servings of grains (bread, cereal, rice, pasta, and other grain foods).
• Eat at least 3 servings of vegetables.
• Eat at least 2 servings of fruit.
• Eat 2 or more servings of low-fat or fat-free dairy products, such as milk, yogurt, or cheese.
• Eat 2 to 3 servings of lean meat, poultry, fish, dried beans, eggs, or nuts.
• Eat a varied diet.
• Eat at least three well-balanced meals.

If any of these options doesn't belong in your day, you may benefit from taking a daily multivitamin and mineral supplement. Supplements are not meant to take the place of any food group or meal, but they can help supplement what you may not get every single day. Your top goal should be to include all of these options as often as possible. If you don't, choose one food group at a time and try to gradually improve your daily eating pattern. Aim to at least eat the minimum number of servings each day.

Other people who may want to consider a multivitamin and mineral supplement include the following:

- Strict vegetarians may need extra calcium, iron, zinc, vitamin B_{12}, and vitamin D.
- Women with heavy menstrual bleeding may need to replace iron each month.
- Women who are pregnant or breastfeeding need more of some nutrients. Be sure to speak with your doctor first.
- Menopausal women can benefit from calcium supplements.
- People on a low-calorie diet can benefit from supplements.
- People over sixty years of age may benefit because they may have a decreased absorption of numerous vitamins and minerals.
- People who suffer from lactose intolerance or milk allergies may be advised to take a vitamin D and a calcium supplement.
- People with impaired nutrient absorption may be instructed by their doctor to take a supplement.
- People who regularly smoke and/or drink alcohol should consider a supplement because these habits could interfere with the body's ability to absorb and use certain vitamins and minerals.

If you feel you are a candidate for a dietary supplement, speak with your doctor or a registered dietitian.

How to Choose a Supplement

If you are going to take a supplement, it is important to take the time to choose the product that is right for you. Follow some of these tips to help you choose a dietary supplement:

- Pick a supplement that contains at least twenty vitamins and minerals essential for good health and no more than 150 percent of the

Reference Daily Intakes (RDI) for each nutrient.

- Choose a supplement tailored to your needs, whether it is age, gender, or medical status.
- Don't be lured by extra ingredients such as choline, inositol, herbs, enzymes, or PABA. These add no proven nutritional benefits and only make them more expensive.
- Check the expiration date on the bottle. If the product is expired, it is not likely to do much good. Vitamins are especially perishable. After the expiration date, they have probably decomposed to the point that they are not very potent.
- Take the supplement only as directed on the bottle or prescribed by your doctor.
- Keep all supplements out of the reach of children.

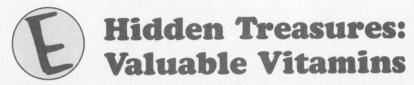

Chapter 6

Hidden Treasures: Valuable Vitamins

A healthy diet consists not only of optimal portions of macronutrients but also recommended levels of essential micronutrients. Micronutrients include vitamins and minerals. It is important to recognize whether you are getting what your body needs and to make necessary changes in your daily diet if you are not.

What Are Vitamins?

Vitamins are natural substances that are necessary for almost every process in the body. Micronutrients help trigger thousands of chemical reactions essential to maintaining good health. Most of these reactions are linked because one triggers another. A missing vitamin or a deficiency of a certain vitamin anywhere in the linked chain can cause a collapse, with health problems being the result.

Vitamins are organic compounds (or compounds that contain carbon) that are required in small amounts and are necessary to promote growth, health, and life. Vitamins are produced by living material such as plants and animals. Most vitamins are not made by the body in sufficient amounts to maintain health so must be obtained through a person's diet. Vitamins are classified into two groups: fat-soluble and water-soluble.

Vitamins are labeled as "micro" nutrients because they are only needed in small amounts to do their jobs properly. Don't let the word "micro" fool you, though; good things come in small packages! The micronutrients are just as essential as the macronutrients in helping to keep your body functioning properly.

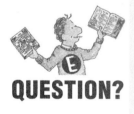

QUESTION?

What are antioxidants?
When cells burn oxygen, they form free radicals. Free radicals can damage body cells, tissue, and DNA, which could lead to the onset of chronic health problems. Certain environmental factors can also cause free radicals. Antioxidants are vitamins that counteract the effects of these harmful free radicals.

Unlike macronutrients, vitamins do not provide calories or supply direct energy, but they do assist the calories in carbohydrates, proteins, and fats to produce energy. Consuming the macronutrients (carbohydrates, proteins, and fat) supplies the thirteen vitamins that the body requires. Vitamins are found in a wide variety of foods, with some foods being better sources than others. For this reason, eating a wide variety of foods ensures a better intake of vitamins.

Dietary Reference Intakes (DRIs)

Before learning why each vitamin is important and how much you need, it is crucial to understand how these values are generated. In the United States, the Food and Nutrition Board of the National Academy of Sciences/National Research Council is responsible for establishing and updating nutrition guidelines. The Recommended Dietary Allowances, or RDAs, have always been the benchmark for adequate nutritional intake in the United States. The RDAs are based on scientific evidence. They reflect the amount of a nutrient that is sufficient to meet the requirement of 97 to 98 percent of healthy individuals in a particular life stage and gender group. Because scientific knowledge of the relationship between nutrition and health has broadened so much, the Food and Nutrition Board partnered with Health Canada in the late 1990s. Together, the agencies developed a new approach called Dietary Reference Intakes (DRIs).

The DRIs represent an approach that serves to optimize health instead of just preventing nutritional deficiencies as the RDAs have. The DRIs include RDAs as goals for intake by individuals but also incorporate three new types of reference values. Where adequate information is available, each nutrient will have a set of DRIs. Each group of nutrients is presently being studied individually. Eventually, DRIs will replace RDAs in the United States and RNIs (Recommended Nutrient Intakes) in Canada.

The DRIs incorporate an average of three types of reference values:

1. Estimated Average Requirement (EAR)
2. Recommended Dietary Allowance (RDA) or Adequate Intake (AI)
3. Tolerable Upper Intake Level (UL)

The DRIs incorporate EAR, which help establish RDAs. The EAR is a daily nutrient intake value that is estimated to meet the requirements of half of the healthy individuals in a life stage and gender group. The RDA is the dietary intake level that is sufficient to meet the nutrient requirements of nearly all (97 to 98 percent) individuals in a specified group. The AIs are a recommended intake value based on observed or experimentally determined estimates of nutrient intake by a group of healthy people that are assumed to be adequate. They are basically used when there is not enough information available to establish an RDA. The Tolerable Upper Intake Level (UL) is the highest daily recommended intake of a nutrient that is unlikely to pose risks of adverse health effects to almost all of the individuals in a specified group.

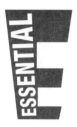

For more information on DRIs, you can contact the U.S. Department of Agriculture's Food and Nutrition Information Center Web site, at *www.nal.usda.gov/fnic.* You can also write to the Food and Nutrition Board at the following address: Institute of Medicine, 500 Fifth Street, NW, Washington, DC 20001.

Fat-Soluble Vitamins

Out of the thirteen vitamins your body needs, four of them are fat-soluble vitamins. These four vitamins are vitamin A, D, E, and K. Fat-soluble vitamins dissolve in fat and are carried throughout your body attached to body chemicals made with fat. This is one important reason you need moderate amounts of fat in your daily diet. The body can store fat-soluble vitamins in its fat stores and in the liver. For this reason, consuming too much of a fat-soluble vitamin, usually in a supplemental form, for a long period of time can be harmful.

Vitamin A

Vitamin A promotes healthy vision (especially night vision), growth and health of cells and tissues, bone growth, and tooth development. Vitamin A also helps protect you from infection by keeping mucous membranes in your mouth, stomach, intestines, respiratory, and urinary tracts healthy. Vitamin A also acts as a powerful antioxidant in the form of beta-carotene.

There are several forms of vitamin A. Retinol is a form that is found in animal foods. It is readily available to the body and is known as preformed vitamin A. Another form of vitamin A is a group called carotenoids, which includes beta-carotene. Beta-carotene is the carotenoid most readily converted by the body to vitamin A. Beta-carotene is found in plant foods that are orange, red, dark yellow, and some that are dark green. These forms are known as building blocks or provitamin forms of vitamin A.

Because vitamin A can be stored in the body, very large intakes over an extended period of time can be harmful. This is only true for preformed vitamin A. Vitamin A toxicity is almost always the result of high supplement intake and not from food. Your body converts beta-carotene to vitamin A only when the body needs it, so beta-carotene is not toxic in any amount. A significant deficiency of vitamin A can cause night blindness and other eye problems, dry and scaly skin, reproductive problems, and poor growth. Too much vitamin A (retinol) can lead to headaches, dry and scaly skin, bone and joint pain, liver damage, vomiting, loss of appetite, abnormal bone growth, nerve damage, and birth defects.

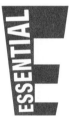

Vitamin A is measured in micrograms for RDA. In supplements and on food labels, it is measured in international units (IU).

When taking a supplement, make sure you are not taking more vitamin A (retinol) than you need for your age range and gender. You will find a breakdown of vitamin A into beta-carotene and retinol on most supplement labels. Even though beta-carotene is not toxic to the body, it is not recommended to take megadoses through supplements. Vitamin A has a UL set at 3,000 micrograms (mcg) or 10,000 IU (international units) per day for adults over eighteen. This is the highest daily recommended intake of vitamin A that is unlikely to pose risks of adverse health effects.

Foods rich in vitamin A (retinol) include beef liver, eggs, milk fortified with vitamin A, other vitamin A–fortified foods, fish oil, margarine, and cheese. Foods rich in vitamin A (beta-carotene) include sweet potatoes, carrots, kale, spinach, apricots, cantaloupe, broccoli, and winter squash.

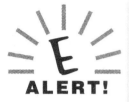

ALERT!

Women who are pregnant should be especially cautioned about taking too much vitamin A through supplements. Studies show that some women who take large doses of vitamin A near the time of conception or early in the pregnancy run a much higher than average risk of delivering an infant with birth defects.

Vitamin D

Vitamin D promotes the absorption and use of two minerals: calcium and phosphorus. It helps deposit these two minerals in bones and teeth, making them stronger and healthier. The body can get vitamin D from two sources—food and the sun. This vitamin is known as the "sunshine vitamin" because the body can make vitamin D after sunlight hits the skin. The body's ability to produce vitamin D from sunlight diminishes with age; therefore, requirements increase for older adults.

Not getting enough vitamin D throughout life can cause osteo-porosis (or brittle bone disease) later in life. Low levels of vitamin D can also increase the risk of bone softening, known as osteoma-lacia, in older adults. A deficiency of vitamin D in children can lead to rickets, or defective bone growth. With the vitamin D fortification of milk, the incidence of rickets has been basically wiped out in the United States.

Because vitamin D is a fat-soluble vitamin, it can be toxic in larger doses. Toxicity can lead to kidney stones or damage, weakened muscles and bones, excessive bleeding, and other health problems. Levels high enough to cause health complications usually come from supplements, not from food or too much sunlight. If you take a supplement that includes vitamin D, make sure it does not contain more than you need for your age range and gender. Vitamin D has a UL set at 50 mcg or 2,000 IU per day for children and adults. There is no UL established for infants.

Foods rich in vitamin D include fortified milk, cheese, egg yolks, salmon, margarine, mackerel, canned sardines, and fortified breakfast cereals.

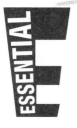

The Adequate Intake (AI) is given in micrograms (mcg) on the Recommended Intake Chart for vitamin D. The vitamin D in supplements and in food is usually measured in international units (IU). The conversion is 1 mcg = 40 IU.

Vitamin E

Vitamin E's main function in promoting health is as a powerful antioxidant. As such, this vitamin helps protect body cells from oxidation, which leads to cell damage. As an antioxidant, vitamin E may affect aging, infertility, heart disease, and cancer. The mineral selenium enhances the antioxidant capabilities of vitamin E. Recent studies have also shown that vitamin E may play a role in reducing muscle inflammation and soreness after vigorous exercise sessions.

Vitamin E is actually a group of substances called tocopherols. All of these tocopherols possess different potencies. For this reason you will often see vitamin E measured in milligrams (mg) of alpha-tocopherol equivalents.

Vitamin E is very abundant in our food supply, so a deficiency is quite rare. Vitamin E is considered nontoxic, even over RDA levels. Vitamin E has a UL set at 1,000 mg per day for adults over eighteen.

Foods rich in vitamin E include dried almonds, vegetable oils, salad dressing, nuts and seeds, wheat germ, peanut butter, and green leafy vegetables.

Vitamin K

Vitamin K's primary function is to help make a protein, known as prothrombin, which is necessary for helping blood to clot. It also aids the body make some other body proteins for blood, bones, and kidneys. Vitamin K is unique in that as well as being obtained from the diet, it is also made in the body, from bacteria in the intestines.

A deficiency of vitamin K is unlikely except for in rare health problems. The prolonged use of antibiotics may tend to cause problems because they destroy some bacteria in your intestines that help to produce vitamin K. There have been no reported problems in ingesting excess amounts of vitamin K, though moderation is still the best policy. Vitamin K has no established UL.

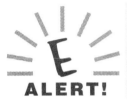

People who take various types of blood-thinning medications or anticoagulants should consume foods containing vitamin K in moderation. If you take these types of medications, ask your doctor about vitamin K intake.

Foods rich in vitamin K include turnip greens, green leafy vegetables like spinach or kale, broccoli, cabbage, beef liver, egg yolk, and wheat bran or wheat germ.

Water-Soluble Vitamins

Unlike the fat-soluble vitamins, water-soluble vitamins dissolve in water. These vitamins are carried in the bloodstream and for the most part are not stored in the body. In general, your body uses what it needs and excretes the rest through urine. For this reason it is important to regularly replenish these vitamins by eating a healthy and varied diet each day. Because water-soluble vitamins dissolve in water, they are much more easily destroyed in cooking and storing than the fat-soluble vitamins.

The water-soluble vitamins consist of the B-complex vitamins and vitamin C. The B vitamins work together in converting carbohydrates, protein, and fats to energy, and many are found in the same foods. For this reason, poor intake of one B vitamin is usually associated with poor intake of other B vitamins.

Thiamine (Vitamin B$_1$)

Thiamine is needed to help produce energy from the carbohydrates that you eat. It also is required for normal functioning of all body cells, especially nerves.

A deficiency of thiamine can lead to beriberi, fatigue, mental confusion, loss of energy, nerve damage, muscle weakness, and impaired growth. Thiamine deficiency is very rare in the United States because most people consume plenty of grain products. Since thiamine is a water-soluble vitamin, the body excretes excess amounts that you consume. There are no known benefits to taking megadoses of thiamine, including the popular belief that it will help boost energy. Thiamine has no established UL.

Foods rich in thiamine (vitamin B$_1$) include whole-grain foods, enriched-grain foods, fortified cereals, beef liver, pork, and wheat germ.

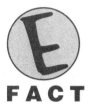

FACT

When whole grains are refined, certain vitamins including the B vitamins are lost during the milling process. Refined grains are therefore enriched, meaning nutrients—including B vitamins—are added back to the grain.

Riboflavin (Vitamin B$_2$)

Just like thiamine, riboflavin plays a key role in releasing energy from the macronutrients to all cells of the body. Riboflavin also helps change the amino acid (building blocks of protein) tryptophan into niacin, another B vitamin. Riboflavin is important in normal growth, production of certain hormones, formation of red blood cells, and in vision and skin health.

A deficiency of riboflavin is unlikely but can cause eye disorders, dry and flaky skin, and burning and dryness of the mouth and tongue. There are no reported problems from consuming too much, but again, moderation is the best policy. Riboflavin has no established UL.

Foods rich in riboflavin (vitamin B$_2$) include beef liver, milk, low-fat yogurt, cheese, enriched-grain foods, whole-grain foods, eggs, and green leafy vegetables.

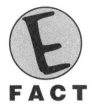

FACT

Riboflavin is easily destroyed by light. For this reason, milk is packaged in opaque plastic or cardboard containers. Riboflavin-rich foods should be stored in darker places and not in transparent containers such as glass.

Niacin (Vitamin B$_3$)

This B vitamin, like its counterparts, is also involved in releasing energy from foods. Niacin specifically helps your body use sugars and fatty acids. In addition, niacin helps enzymes function normally in the body and promotes health of nerves, skin, and the digestive system.

Although niacin deficiency is rare among populations that eat adequate amounts of protein-rich foods, it can cause pellagra. Symptoms include diarrhea, mental confusion, and skin problems. Niacin, in large doses, has been used as a cholesterol-lowering supplement. Because large doses can cause symptoms such as flushed skin, rashes, and even liver damage, this should only be done under doctors' supervision. Niacin has a UL set at 35 mg per day for adults over eighteen.

Niacin is usually measured in niacin equivalents (NE) because it comes from two sources: niacin itself and from the amino acid tryptophan. Tryptophan can be converted to niacin in the presence of riboflavin and of vitamin B$_6$.

Foods rich in niacin include meat, poultry, fish, legumes, peanut butter, enriched- and fortified-grain products, and yogurt.

Pyridoxine (Vitamin B$_6$)

Vitamin B$_6$ is necessary in helping your body to make nonessential amino acids (the building blocks of protein). These nonessential amino acids are used to make necessary body cells. Vitamin B$_6$ also helps to turn the amino acid tryptophan into niacin and serotonin (a messenger in the brain). This vitamin also helps produce insulin, hemoglobin, and antibodies that help fight infection.

Deficiency symptoms of vitamin B_6 include depression, nausea, and greasy and flaky skin. In infants, a deficiency can cause irritability and mental convulsions in severe cases. Proper amounts of breast milk and properly prepared infant formulas contain enough of this vitamin to protect against deficiencies. Vitamin B_6 is one of the few water-soluble vitamins that can cause harm if taken in megadoses. Large doses taken over a long period can damage the nervous system. Vitamin B_6 has a UL set at 100 mg per day for adults over eighteen.

Foods rich in vitamin B_6 include protein-rich foods, such as chicken, fish, pork, liver, peanut butter, whole grains, nuts, and legumes.

Cobalamin (Vitamin B_{12})

Vitamin B_{12} works closely with folic acid to form red blood cells. It also helps maintain the nervous system and is essential for the normal functioning of all body cells. Vitamin B_{12} is necessary in assisting the body to use fat and some amino acids.

A deficiency of vitamin B_{12} can result in anemia, fatigue, nerve damage, smooth tongue, and very sensitive skin. It is important to know that a deficiency of this vitamin can be hidden, and even progress, if extra folic acid is taken to treat or prevent anemia.

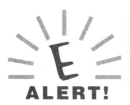

ALERT!

Since B_{12} is found mostly in animal products, strict vegetarians and infants are at risk of developing a B_{12} deficiency. Including fortified foods and/or dietary supplements daily can help prevent this.

The classic deficiency symptom of vitamin B_{12} is anemia. This vitamin cannot be absorbed without the help of a substance called the intrinsic factor. Because this intrinsic factor is made in the lining of the stomach, the elderly and people with gastrointestinal disorders may not absorb the vitamin B_{12} their body needs. There are also people who, for either medical or genetic reasons, are missing this intrinsic factor. This problem can usually be treated with B_{12} injections. When anemia is caused by a lack of the intrinsic factor, it is called pernicious anemia. When the anemia is caused by poor dietary intake, it is called macrocytic anemia. Because of the body's ability to store vitamin B_{12} and because of the small amount needed daily, a deficiency can take years to develop. There are no known toxic effects of taking large doses of vitamin B_{12}, but neither is there any scientific evidence that extra vitamin B_{12} helps boost energy. Vitamin B_{12} has no established UL.

Foods rich in vitamin B_{12} include meat, fish, poultry, eggs, milk and other dairy foods, and fortified foods.

Folic Acid (Folacin or Folate)

Folic acid's main role is to maintain the cell's genetic code—DNA, the master plan for cell reproduction. It also works with vitamin B_{12} to form hemoglobin in red blood cells.

In recent years, folic acid has gained much attention for its role in reducing the risk for neural tube birth defects, such as spina bifida, in newborn babies. The embryo's neural tube is what becomes the spinal cord. It is vital that pregnant women or women of childbearing years consume enough folic acid through food and supplements, especially during the first trimester. Other deficiencies of folic acid include anemia, impaired growth, and abnormal digestive function. Taking too much folic acid through supplements can mask a vitamin B_{12} deficiency and could interfere with other medications. In the synthetic form—the form used to fortify foods and in supplements—folic acid has a UL of 1,000 mcg per day for adults over eighteen.

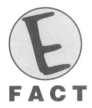

FACT

Most enriched-grain products now have to be fortified with folic acid, according to a new FDA regulation. This is to help ensure that women get enough folic acid to help prevent neural tube birth defects during pregnancy.

Foods rich in folic acid include some fruits, such as oranges, as well as leafy vegetables, legumes, liver, wheat germ, some fortified cereals, avocados, and enriched-grain products.

Biotin

Biotin participates in the metabolism of the macronutrients for energy and helps your body produce energy in the cells. For people who eat a healthy, well-balanced diet, deficiency is not a problem. In the rare cases when deficiency does occur, symptoms include heart abnormalities, loss of appetite, fatigue, depression, and dry skin. Biotin has no known toxic effects and no established UL.

This vitamin is found in a wide variety of foods, such as eggs, liver, yeast breads, cereals, wheat germ, and oatmeal.

Pantothenic Acid

Like biotin, pantothenic acid also participates in the metabolism of the macronutrients for energy and helps your body produce energy in the cells. In addition, pantothenic acid functions in the production of some hormones and neurotransmitters in the brain.

Deficiency is again rare in those eating a healthy, well-balanced diet. When deficiency does occur, symptoms include nausea, fatigue, and difficulty sleeping. The only possible effects of consuming too much pantothenic acid are occasional diarrhea and water retention. Pantothenic acid has no established UL.

Foods rich in pantothenic acid include meat, poultry, fish, whole-grain cereals, legumes, yogurt, sweet potatoes, milk, and eggs.

Vitamin C (Ascorbic Acid)

Vitamin C is often associated with warding off the common cold. There is no conclusive data that large doses of vitamin C prevent colds; they may reduce the severity or duration of symptoms, but there is no definitive evidence. Scientific evidence does not suggest taking large doses of vitamin C on a regular basis to boost immunity or to decrease risks for the common cold.

But vitamin C does have some very important functions. Vitamin C produces collagen, a connective tissue that holds muscles, bones, and other tissues together. It also helps form and repair red blood cells, bones, and other tissue; helps protect you from bruising by keeping capillary walls and blood vessels firm; helps keep your gums healthy; helps heal cuts and wounds; and helps keep your immune system strong and healthy. Vitamin C helps your body absorb iron from plant sources, which is not as easily absorbed as iron from animal foods. Vitamin C is one of the very powerful antioxidants. As an antioxidant, vitamin C attacks free radicals in the body's fluids.

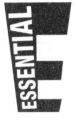

Cigarette smokers need at least twice as much vitamin C as nonsmokers, that is, at least 100 milligrams per day.

Since vitamin C is so widely available in our foods, deficiency is rare. Possible deficiency symptoms include poor wound healing, higher susceptibility to infections, bleeding gums, hemorrhaging, and, in severe cases, scurvy. Scurvy is a disease characterized by bleeding and swollen gums, joint pain, muscle wasting, and bruising.

Because vitamin C is a water-soluble vitamin, your body excretes the excess that may be consumed. Very large doses, though, could cause kidney stones, nausea, and diarrhea. The effects of taking large amounts over extended periods of time are not yet known. Vitamin C has a UL set at 2,000 mg per day for adults over eighteen.

Most fruits and vegetables are great sources of vitamin C. These include all citrus fruits, berries, melons, peppers, dark green leafy vegetables, potatoes (especially the skin), and tomatoes.

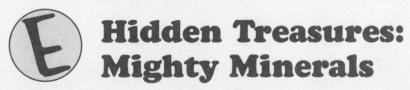

Chapter 7

Hidden Treasures: Mighty Minerals

A balanced diet means getting all of the minerals, as well as vitamins, that your body needs to maintain good health. The best way to guarantee optimal intake of minerals is to understand why these nutrients are important and to learn how to design and consume a nutritious, balanced diet based on your individual needs.

What Are Minerals?

Minerals are different from vitamins in that they do not contain carbon. This makes them inorganic compounds. They cannot be destroyed as easily as vitamins by heat or poor handling. Minerals are involved in a variety of functions in the body. They help to both regulate body processes and give your body structure. Just like vitamins, minerals are only needed in small amounts.

All minerals are absorbed into your intestines and then are transported and stored in your body in various ways. Some minerals pass directly into your bloodstream, which transports them to the cells; the excess passes out of the body through the urine. Other minerals, such as calcium, attach to proteins and become part of your body structure (in the case of calcium, the bones). Because these types of minerals are stored, large amounts taken for a long period of time can be harmful.

More than sixty minerals are found in the body. Of those, twenty-two are considered essential to good health. Minerals are divided into two categories: major and trace. As the names imply, major minerals are required in larger amounts than trace.

Potassium

Potassium is an electrolyte that works closely with its counterparts, chloride and sodium. Over 95 percent of potassium is in the body's cells. Potassium helps regulate the flow of fluids and minerals in and out of the body's cells. It also helps maintain normal blood pressure, maintain heart and kidney function, and transmit nerve impulses and contraction of muscles. Potassium is very important in converting blood sugar into glycogen, the storage form of blood sugar in your muscles and liver. A potassium shortage in the muscles can produce great fatigue and muscle weakness.

A potassium deficiency is unlikely for most healthy people because this mineral is so widely available in foods. Deficiency could occur as a result of chronic diarrhea, vomiting, diabetic acidosis, kidney disease, or prolonged use of laxatives or diuretics. Symptoms of potassium deficiency include weakness, loss of appetite, nausea, and fatigue.

Most people can handle excess potassium because it is excreted in the urine. If the excess cannot be excreted—for instance, in the case of someone with kidney disease—it can cause heart problems. These people will most likely be advised by their doctors to limit foods containing potassium.

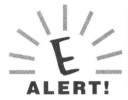

ALERT!

If you need to limit your potassium content, be aware that salt substitutes contain potassium chloride instead of the sodium chloride that is in table salt.

There is no RDA or DRI for potassium, but the minimum amount suggested for adults is 2,000 milligrams per day. Some experts recommend a higher intake, around 3,500 milligrams per day, to help protect against high blood pressure.

Potassium is found in a wide range of foods but especially in fruits and vegetables as well as in fresh meat, poultry, and fish. It is important to have a proper balance of both potassium and sodium in the diet. Studies have indicated a possible link between a diet high in sodium and low in potassium with an increased risk of cancer, heart disease, high blood pressure, and stroke. On the other hand, a diet high in potassium and low in sodium may help to protect or decrease the risk for these health problems.

Sodium

Sodium is also an electrolyte that works closely with potassium and chloride. In contrast to potassium, most of the body's sodium is found outside the cells in blood and other body fluids. There is a pump in the membrane of all cells that flushes sodium out of and brings potassium into the cell. If sodium is not pumped out properly, water accumulates in the cell, causing it to swell.

Sodium helps regulate the movement of body fluids in and out of cells. It also helps relax your muscles (including your heart muscle), transmit nerve impulses, and regulate blood pressure. Sodium can contribute to hypertension by raising blood pressure.

A sodium deficiency is unlikely except in cases of prolonged diarrhea, vomiting, fasting, starvation, or kidney problems. Symptoms can include nausea, dizziness, dehydration, muscle weakness, loss of appetite, and muscle cramps.

Healthy people excrete excess sodium. In the United States, the typical diet contains excessive amounts of sodium. Processed foods are one of the biggest contributors to our sodium intake. The rest comes from table salt and small amounts that occur naturally in foods. There is no RDA or DRI for sodium; however, the amount considered safe and adequate is 500 milligrams daily. Healthy American adults should reduce their sodium intake to no more than 2,400 milligrams per day. This is almost 1¼ teaspoons of sodium chloride or table salt each day.

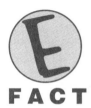

FACT

The American Heart Association says that "reducing the amount of sodium you consume may help you reduce or avoid high blood pressure."

Chloride

Chloride is another electrolyte that works closely with potassium and sodium. Chloride also helps regulate body fluids in and out of body cells. Chloride joins sodium in surrounding the fluids outside the cells. This mineral is a component of stomach acid that helps with the digestion of food and the absorption of nutrients. Chloride also helps to transmit nerve impulses.

A deficiency of chloride is rare since salt, which is made of sodium chloride, is such a large part of the typical American diet. The deficiency symptoms of chloride are similar to that of sodium. As stated earlier, many salt substitutes also contain chloride in the form of potassium chloride.

Magnesium

Every cell in the body needs magnesium. Magnesium is a requirement for more than 300 body enzymes, body chemicals that regulate all kinds of body functions. This mineral helps maintain normal nerve and muscle function, keeps heart rhythm steady, and helps keep bones strong.

Magnesium is involved in energy metabolism and protein production.

Magnesium deficiency is rare in the United States. When magnesium deficiency does occur, it is usually due to excessive loss of magnesium in urine, gastrointestinal system disorders that cause a loss of magnesium or limit magnesium absorption, or a chronically low intake of magnesium. Deficiency can also result from an increase in urine output—like that caused by diuretics—poorly controlled diabetes, and alcoholism. Symptoms can include irregular heartbeat, nausea, weakness, and mental confusion.

Too much magnesium is not harmful unless the mineral is not excreted properly due to disorders such as kidney disease. Signs of excess magnesium include mental status changes, nausea, diarrhea, appetite loss, muscle weakness, difficulty breathing, extremely low blood pressure, and irregular heartbeat. The UL for magnesium is 350 mg per day for adults over eighteen. Magnesium can be found in a wide variety of foods. The best sources include legumes, nuts, avocados, wheat germ, and whole grains. Green vegetables can be good sources too.

Phosphorus

Phosphorus is second only to calcium in terms of its abundance in the body. Phosphorus contributes to the structure of bones and teeth. It helps generate energy in every cell in the body and acts as the main regulator in converting dietary carbohydrate, protein, and fat to energy. Phosphorus is vital to growth, maintenance, and repair of all body tissue. This mineral is also a component of many proteins. It helps activate B vitamins and is a component of the storage form of energy in the body.

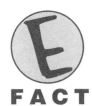

FACT

Soft drinks contain as much as 500 milligrams phosphoric acid, which can contribute to excessive intakes if consumed regularly.

A deficiency of phosphorus is very rare. However, absorption can be reduced by the long-term and excessive use of antacids containing aluminum hydroxide, increasing the risk of deficiency. Symptoms can include bone loss, weakness, loss of appetite, and pain.

Too much phosphorus can lower the level of calcium in the blood, which can really be a problem if calcium intake is already low in the diet. This can result in increased bone loss and an increased risk for osteoporosis, or brittle bone disease.

Phosphorus is found in almost all food groups. The best sources are protein-rich foods like milk, meat, poultry, fish, and eggs. Legumes and nuts are also good sources. Whole grains can also be good sources of phosphorus.

Phosphorus has a daily UL set at 4 grams for adults aged eighteen to seventy, 3 grams for adults over seventy, 3.5 grams for pregnant women, and 4 grams for breastfeeding women.

Calcium

Calcium is one of the most abundant minerals in the body. The average healthy adult male body contains about 2 to 3 pounds of calcium; the average healthy female body contains about 2 pounds. Of course this amount depends on body composition, the size of the body frame, bone density, and on how much bone has been lost through the aging process. About 99 percent of the body's calcium is in the bones. The remaining 1 percent is found in body fluids and other cells.

Calcium's primary function is to help build and maintain bones and teeth. In addition, calcium helps blood clot, helps your muscles contract and your heart beat, helps regulate blood pressure, plays a role in normal nerve function and nerve transmission, and helps regulate the secretion of hormones and digestive enzymes. Calcium works in conjunction with vitamin D, phosphorus, and fluoride to help promote strong and healthy bones. Vitamin D is necessary for the absorption of calcium in the body.

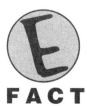

FACT

A constant supply of calcium is needed throughout life especially during growth spurts in childhood, during pregnancy, and while breastfeeding. But these are not the only times calcium is needed. It is important to get adequate calcium throughout your life.

Low levels of calcium intake can lead to osteomalacia (softening of the bones) and an increased risk of osteoporosis. A deficiency in children can interfere with growth. Even a mild deficiency throughout a lifetime can lead to a loss of bone and bone density. A decreased intake of calcium can also contribute to muscle spasms and leg cramps as well as high blood pressure.

Calcium has a UL set at 2,500 mg per day for adults and children. No UL is established for infants. When consuming supplements up to this amount, no adverse effects are likely. However, higher doses over an extended period of time may cause kidney stones and poor kidney function as well as reduce the absorption of other minerals such as iron and zinc.

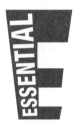

Label claims on food packages can tell you a lot about the vitamins and minerals they contain. The terms "high," "rich in," and "excellent source of" mean the food has 20 percent or more of the daily value. The terms "good source," "contains," or "provides" mean 10 to 19 percent of the daily value is provided. And the terms "more," "enriched," "fortified," or "added" mean the food provides 10 percent or more of the daily value.

Some of the best sources of calcium are foods in the dairy group, such as milk, cheese, and yogurt. In addition, some dark green leafy vegetables, such as broccoli, spinach, kale, and collards, are also good sources. Other good sources include fish with edible bones, such as sardines and salmon, as well as calcium-fortified soymilk, tofu made with calcium, shelled almonds, cooked dried beans, calcium-fortified cereals, and calcium-fortified orange juice.

Trace Minerals

Minerals that are needed in smaller amounts than the major minerals are referred to as trace minerals or trace elements. Even though our bodies only require a small amount of these minerals, they are still very important to proper health. Most trace minerals are needed in amounts of less than 20 mg per day.

Other trace minerals include arsenic, silicon, vanadium, nickel, and boron. Little is known about these trace elements and their role in human health. In fact, there are no RDAs, DRIs, or safe and adequate ranges set for these minerals because not enough is known about what the body requires for proper health and functioning. A healthy, varied, and balanced diet is the best way to ensure you consume safe and adequate amounts of these other trace minerals.

Zinc

Almost every cell in the body contains zinc, and it is also part of over 70 different types of enzymes. Zinc is known as the second most abundant trace mineral in the body. It is essential for normal growth and development and is vital to a healthy immune system. Zinc assists the body in using the macronutrients (carbohydrates, proteins, and fats). In addition, zinc functions in the production of proteins, proper functioning of the hormone insulin, the maintenance of your genetic code, and normal taste.

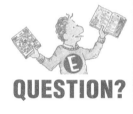

QUESTION?

Is it helpful to take over-the-counter zinc lozenges when you feel the symptoms of a cold coming on?
Scientists have found that in test tubes, zinc can prevent cold viruses from reproducing themselves. But as for its ability to fight the disease in the human body, the jury is still out. Some studies have showed that if zinc lozenges are taken within twenty-four hours of coming down with cold symptoms, they may help shorten the length of the cold.

Adequate levels of zinc are vital to good health because zinc is involved in so many enzyme and body functions. A deficiency of zinc in childhood can cause retarded growth; during pregnancy, deficiency can cause birth defects. Other deficiency symptoms include loss of appetite, skin changes, and reduced resistance to infection. Too much zinc, especially from supplements, can trigger harmful side effects that include impaired copper absorption. The UL for zinc is 40 mg per day for adults over eighteen years of age.

Good food sources of zinc include animal foods such as meat, seafood, and liver. Milk and eggs supply a little less zinc. Foods such as whole-grain products, wheat germ, legumes, nuts, and seeds have a good concentration of zinc; however, the zinc that plant foods provide is less available to the body.

Iodine

Iodine is a component of the thyroid hormone called thyroxin. Thyroxin regulates the rate at which the body burns calories or uses energy from food. With a deficiency of iodine, the body cannot make sufficient amounts of thyroxin. As a result, the rate at which the body burns calories slows down. A deficiency can be especially harmful in pregnant women, the developing fetus, and the newborn. Poor iodine intake is associated with hypothyroidism and/or the development of an enlarged thyroid gland, commonly called a goiter. Too much iodine can also cause the development of a goiter, but this is not common at the levels that are consumed on average in the United States. Iodine has a UL set at 1,100 mcg per day for adults over eighteen.

Iodine is found naturally in saltwater fish and seafood such as seaweeds. Most of the iodine in the United States is ingested through the form of iodized salt.

Selenium

Selenium works with vitamin E as an antioxidant. Together, they help protect cells from damaging free radicals that may lead to health problems such as cancer and heart disease. Selenium is also important in cell growth.

A severe deficiency, although extremely rare, is associated with a severe heart disorder. The body only requires a small amount of selenium. Too much selenium over prolonged periods of time can produce signs of toxicity that can be harmful. Selenium has a UL set at 400 mcg per day for adults over eighteen. A normal healthy diet with a variety of foods generally provides the selenium required for normal body function. Food sources of selenium include seafood, liver, and kidney, as well as other meats. Many plant foods contain selenium, such as grain products and seeds, but the amount is directly related to the level of selenium in the soil that produces the food. Most fruits and vegetables don't contain much.

Copper

Copper is found in all the tissues in the body but is concentrated in the brain, heart, kidney, and liver. Copper is the third most abundant essential trace mineral, after iron and zinc. Copper helps the body make hemoglobin (needed to carry oxygen to red blood cells) and red blood cells by aiding in the absorption of iron in the body. Copper is part of many enzymes in the body and helps produce energy in cells. In addition, copper helps make hormones that regulate a variety of body functions, including heartbeat, blood pressure, and wound healing.

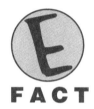

FACT

A copper deficiency can cause iron deficiency since copper is required for proper iron absorption and utilization.

Copper deficiency rarely comes from the diet. Most deficiencies are due to a genetic problem or from too much zinc. Copper toxicity is rare. High daily intakes can cause nausea and vomiting. Copper has a UL set at 10,000 mcg per day for adults over eighteen.

Copper is found mostly in organ meats, especially liver, and in seafood, nuts, and seeds. It can also be found in poultry, legumes, and dark green leafy vegetables. Cooking in copper pots increases the copper content of foods.

Manganese

Manganese serves as part of many types of enzymes including enzymes involved in blood sugar control, energy metabolism, and thyroid hormone function. Manganese is widely distributed in food, so deficiencies are very rare. Deficiencies could be associated with impaired fertility, growth retardation, birth defects, and general weakness. Consuming harmful levels of manganese is also rare. Too much, though, could inhibit the absorption of iron, copper, and zinc. Manganese has a

UL set at 11 mg per day for adults over eighteen. Manganese is found mostly in whole-grain foods, along with some fruits and vegetables.

Fluoride

Fluoride helps to harden tooth enamel and protect your teeth from decay. When the diet is adequate in fluoride, bones are stronger and more resistant to degeneration and osteoporosis, or brittle bone disease. Fluoride works with calcium, phosphorus, magnesium, and vitamin D to form and maintain healthy bones and teeth. A deficiency of fluoride can lead to weakened tooth enamel and a higher incidence of dental caries. Too much fluoride can cause mottling, pitting, dulling, and staining of the teeth. Fluoride has a UL set at 10 mg per day for adults over eighteen.

The primary means of obtaining fluoride is drinking and/or cooking with fluoridated water. Fluoride is not widely available in foods, but it can be found in tea, especially if made with fluoridated water, and fish with edible bones, such as canned salmon.

Chromium

Chromium works closely with insulin to help your body use blood sugar or glucose. Without chromium, the action of insulin is blocked and blood sugar levels elevate. Chromium is critical to proper maintenance of blood sugar.

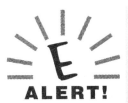
ALERT!

A very popular supplement in the weight-loss world is chromium picolinate, which many manufacturers claim will help to improve your body's lean-to-fat ratio. Chromium picolinate is simply a form of the mineral chromium. Taking megadoses of any supplement is not recommended. Talk to your doctor if you are considering taking chromium picolinate supplements.

The primary sign of a chromium deficiency is intolerance to glucose, which leads to high blood sugar and insulin levels. This can sometimes look like diabetes. Consuming too much from dietary sources is unlikely. There is no UL established for chromium at this time. Trivalent chromium, the form in most chromium supplements, is extremely safe. The best sources of chromium include meats, eggs, cheese, and whole-grain foods.

Molybdenum

Molybdenum works with riboflavin to help form the body's iron into hemoglobin for making red blood cells. Molybdenum functions as a component of many different enzymes. With a normal diet there is no worry of deficiency because this mineral is needed in such small amounts. Too much molybdenum can interfere with the body's ability to use copper. Molybdenum has a UL set at 2,200 mcg per day for adults over eighteen. Molybdenum is found mostly in milk, legumes, bread, and grain products.

Iron

Iron is the mineral that occurs in the greatest amount in the blood. Almost two-thirds of the iron in your body is found in hemoglobin, the protein in red blood cells that carries oxygen to your body's tissues. Smaller amounts of iron are found in myoglobin, a protein that helps supply oxygen to muscle and contributes to the color of muscle. About 15 percent of your body's iron is stored for future needs and activated when dietary intake is inadequate. The remainder is in your body's tissues as part of proteins that help your body function. Iron is also needed for a strong immune system and for energy production.

In the United States, iron deficiency is one of the most common nutrient deficiencies. Iron deficiency can lead to anemia, fatigue, and infections. Anemia, the last stage of iron deficiency, is a condition in which the blood is deficient in red blood cells or the hemoglobin (iron-containing) portion of red blood cells. Symptoms include extreme fatigue due to the lack of oxygen being delivered to needed tissues. Iron is the most common though not the sole cause of anemia.

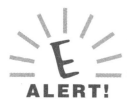

If you feel you are a candidate for possible iron deficiency or you feel you may have symptoms, talk with your doctor about testing your iron stores before self-prescribing a supplement.

Certain types of people are at higher risk for iron deficiency and should be screened periodically:

- Infants and children, because of their growth and choosy eating habits.
- Adolescents, especially girls who have started their menstrual cycle, who consume a junk food diet.
- Women who are pregnant, because they are supporting their needs as well as the baby's.
- The elderly population because of poor dietary intake and decreased iron absorption due to aging.
- Women of childbearing age who experience excessive menstrual bleeding, because they are losing iron-rich blood each month.
- Strict vegetarians who eat only plant foods, because the iron in these foods is not absorbed as well as the iron in animal products.
- People who abuse crash diets and people suffering from eating disorders, because there is a good chance they are not meeting their requirements for iron.
- A person who loses an excessive amount of blood through surgery or other incident.

Iron deficiency can occur from decreased dietary intake, increased need for iron, blood loss, diminished iron absorption or utilization, or a combination of these factors.

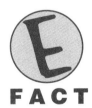

FACT

Women who are menopausal and postmenopausal have a decreased need for iron.

Your body usually maintains normal iron status by controlling the amount of iron absorbed from food, but iron can build up and become harmful in people who have a genetic disorder called hemochromatosis. This disorder, which usually occurs in men, causes excessive iron to accumulate in soft tissue. The result can be heart problems and other abnormalities. In children, large amounts of iron can have serious consequences. Keep iron supplements and other adult nutrient supplements out of the reach of children. Children should get immediate medical attention if they take an overdose of iron supplements.

Iron supplementation may be indicated when an iron deficiency is diagnosed and when diet alone cannot restore bodily iron content to normal levels within an acceptable time frame.

Taking iron supplements can cause side effects such as nausea, vomiting, constipation, diarrhea, dark colored stools, and/or abdominal distress. To minimize these side effects, take the supplement in divided doses and with food. It is best to seek the advice of your doctor before taking an iron supplement. Iron has a UL set at 45 mg per day for adults over eighteen.

Table 7-1 Food Sources of Iron	
Good sources of heme iron	**Good sources of nonheme iron**
Beef liver	Fortified breakfast cereals
Lean red meats	Nuts and seeds
Poultry	Bran
Pork	Spinach
Salmon	Legumes
Lamb	Lentils
Veal	Dried fruit
	Egg yolk (exception to the rule)
	Whole-wheat bread
	Wheat germ
	Enriched rice, cooked

Iron is contained in foods of both plant and animal origin. The iron in plant foods is called nonheme iron and is not absorbed as well as the iron from animal foods, called heme iron. Consuming vitamin C–rich foods at meals can help enhance your body's ability to absorb nonheme iron. This is especially important for strict vegetarians who do not eat animal foods. Grain products, cereals, and flours that are enriched or fortified with iron are good dietary sources of nonheme iron. The improved iron status of millions of infants, children, and women has been attributed to the addition of iron to infant formula, cereals, and grain products.

Chapter 8

Two Nutrition Wonders: Fiber and Water

Fiber and water are two forgotten nutrients that are essential to a healthy diet. The more you learn about why both of these nutrients are so important to good health, the more you will be motivated to permanently include them in your daily life.

Focus on Fiber

Fiber is exclusively found in plant foods. It's a part of plants that our body cannot digest, the part that gives a plant its shape and structure. Dietary fiber is called a complex carbohydrate, but because it cannot be digested or absorbed into the bloodstream, it is not considered a nutrient. Basically fiber comes in and goes out of the body. However, it does some pretty amazing things on its travels.

Fiber fits into two categories, soluble and insoluble, each with its own health benefits. What differentiates them is that soluble fiber dissolves in water and insoluble does not. Some foods contain predominantly one type of fiber; others contain both types. The key is eating a variety of fiber-rich foods every day that will provide you with the health benefits of both soluble and insoluble fiber.

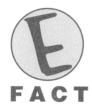

FACT

Currently, the dietary fiber intake among adults in the United States averages about 15 grams. That's about half the recommended amount.

Soluble fibers naturally found in plants include gums, mucilages, psyllium, and pectins. Foods that contain these fibers include peas, beans, oats, barley, and some fruits (especially apples with skin, oranges, prunes, strawberries, and bananas) and some vegetables (especially carrots, broccoli, and cauliflower). Because soluble fiber dissolves in liquids, it is added to foods for its gummy or viscous properties. It is used in some low-fat and fat-free foods to add texture and consistency. Soluble fiber binds to fatty substances and promotes their excretion, which in turn seems to help lower blood cholesterol levels. The American Heart Association says, "When eaten regularly as part of a low-fat, low-cholesterol diet, soluble fiber has been shown to help lower blood cholesterol." Soluble fibers also help to slow the absorption of glucose (or blood sugar), which in turn helps to control blood sugar levels.

Insoluble fiber is known as "roughage." Insoluble fibers give plants their structure. The types found in plants include cellulose, hemicellulose, and lignin. Foods that contain these fibers include whole-wheat products, wheat bran, corn bran, some fruits (especially the skin), and many vegetables including cauliflower, green beans, potatoes with skin, and broccoli. Insoluble fibers do not dissolve in water, but they hold onto water as they move waste through your intestinal tract. By holding on to water, they add bulk and softness to the stool and therefore promote regularity and help prevent constipation. Insoluble fibers also help accelerate intestinal transit time, decreasing the time that waste is in the colon. This is the time that potentially harmful substances in food waste linger in the intestines.

Fiber's Health Benefits

Studies show that a diet rich in fiber as part of a varied, balanced, and low-fat eating pattern may help prevent some chronic diseases. No matter how good your present health is, you can certainly benefit from adding more fiber to your diet. Fiber not only promotes health, it may also help reduce the risk for digestive problems, heart disease, some types of cancer, and diabetes. A fiber-rich diet can also help to promote weight loss.

Digestive Health

One digestive health benefit mentioned above is that insoluble fibers help with proper bowel function by drawing water into the digestive tract. Insoluble fiber also helps to move waste quickly through the colon. This accelerated transit time and increased bulk may help prevent hemorrhoids, constipation, and diverticulosis. Thousands of Americans have diverticulosis (a condition of the colon), but unless the diverticula become inflamed, they may not realize it. This condition can be aggravated by a diet that is too low in fiber. Too little bulk in the intestine can increase pressure in the colon. As a result, little pouches—or diverticula—form in the colon walls. These pouches in turn can collect food and become infected and inflamed. Eating a diet rich in fiber can reduce this pressure and help to prevent these pouches from forming.

Heart Disease

The ability of a fiber-rich diet to help lower blood cholesterol levels can help decrease the risk of heart disease. Soluble fibers may help to lower blood cholesterol levels, especially LDL-cholesterol (the bad cholesterol), which if high is a major risk factor for heart disease. It seems that fiber also helps bile acids, which are made of cholesterol, to pass through the intestines as waste. This in turn seems to assist the body in absorbing less dietary cholesterol. The best way to lower total and LDL-cholesterol is to eat a fiber-rich diet and reduce intake of saturated fat and cholesterol. In obese persons, weight reduction can also significantly reduce cholesterol.

Cancer

Along with a healthy diet, a fiber-rich diet may decrease the risk of colon and rectal cancer. With the accelerated transit time, the digestive tract's exposure to carcinogens (cancer-causing agents) is minimized. Fiber may also bind with harmful bacteria and transport them out of the body. A high-fiber diet is also linked to a reduced risk of breast cancer. This is basically because foods higher in fiber are usually lower in fat and calories, two risk factors associated with breast and other cancers. The association between fiber and cancer risk is inconclusive, but eating high-fiber foods is still recommended. They contain other substances that can help prevent cancer, and they have other health benefits besides.

Diabetes

A diet that is high in fiber, especially soluble fiber, may be helpful for people with diabetes. By helping control blood sugar levels, soluble fibers could reduce the needed amount of insulin or medication. We don't yet know how soluble fibers help lower blood sugar levels. It may be because fiber increases the emptying time of the stomach, which could help slow down the absorption of sugar into the bloodstream. Because it is not yet fully understood, people with diabetes should follow the same guidelines related to fiber and a healthful diet as the general population.

If you have diabetes and want to use more soluble fiber in controlling your blood sugar, talk to your health-care provider or dietitian.

Weight Loss

Because fiber-rich foods are often lower in fat and calories, a fiber-rich diet may also help you watch your waistline. Fiber-rich foods also take longer to chew, which can slow down your eating and help you to eat less. The added bulk of fiber-rich foods can help make you feel fuller longer after eating and help decrease the need to nibble too soon after a meal. This does not mean you will lose weight from eating fiber, but it does mean that eating foods higher in fiber will assist your weight loss efforts. As with all of the health benefits associated with a fiber-rich diet, it is important to incorporate it with a lower fat intake and an active lifestyle.

Are You Getting Enough Fiber?

The amount of total dietary fiber you should consume each day is about 25 to 35 grams from food, not supplements (unless recommended by your doctor). There is no RDA for total fiber intake, but the aim should be to consume fiber daily from both soluble and insoluble fibers from a wide variety of foods.

You don't need to eat huge amounts of plant foods to get your total fiber needs for the day. Your everyday food choices can supply all that you need. If you eat at least five servings of fruits and vegetables and three servings of whole grains each day, you will come very close to the amount of fiber you need.

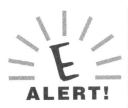

ALERT!

You can overdo it on fiber. Eating more than 50 to 60 grams of fiber per day may cause a decrease in the amount of vitamins and minerals—such as zinc, iron, magnesium, and calcium—that your body absorbs. Large amounts can also cause gas, diarrhea, and bloating.

Boost Your Fiber Intake

When increasing your fiber intake, do it gradually over a number of days or even weeks to allow your body time to adjust to the changes. Adding fiber too quickly can result in uncomfortable symptoms such as gas, diarrhea, cramping, and bloating. When increasing your intake of fiber, it is also important to increase your water and fluid intake. Increasing your fluids helps the fiber to move more easily through your intestines and can help prevent constipation. Aim to drink at least eight 8-ounce glasses of fluids a day.

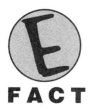

Children need fiber also but not as much as adults. Fiber can fill children up quickly, making it difficult for them to eat other nutritious foods. Estimate the number of grams a child should have each day by adding 5 to the child's age. For example, a seven-year-old child should have 12 grams (7 + 5) of fiber each day.

Adding fiber to your diet may be easier than you think. Here are some tips that can help you get started:

- Look at the fiber content on the Nutrition Facts Label on packaged foods. Good sources of fiber have at least 2.5 grams of fiber per serving.
- Try substituting higher fiber foods, such as whole-grain breads, brown rice, whole-wheat pasta, and fruits and vegetables, for lower fiber foods, such as white bread, white rice, candy, and chips.
- Eat more raw vegetables and fresh fruits, and include the skins when appropriate. Cooking vegetables can reduce their fiber content, and skins are a good source of fiber.
- Plan to eat high-fiber foods such as fruits, vegetables, legumes, or whole-grain starches at every meal.
- Start your day with a high-fiber breakfast cereal, such as bran cereal or oatmeal. Look for cereals that contain at least 5 grams of fiber per serving.

- Add fresh fruit to your cereal for an extra fiber boost.
- Eat a variety of high-fiber foods to ensure you get a mix of both types of fiber.
- Use snacks to increase your fiber intake by nibbling on higher fiber foods, such as dried fruits, popcorn, fresh fruit, raw vegetables, or whole-wheat crackers.
- Try to eat legumes, or dried beans, at least two to three times per week. Add them to salads, soups, casseroles, or spaghetti sauce.
- Eat whole fruits more often than juice. Most of the fiber in fruit is found in the skin and pulp, which is removed when the juice is made.

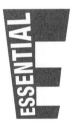

Just because bread says "wheat" or because it is brown in color does not mean it is high in fiber or that it has fiber at all. The key words to look for are "whole wheat" or "whole grain." On average, a slice of whole-wheat bread has 2 to 3 grams of fiber.

Fiber Label Lingo

The food label on packaged foods lists fiber in grams per serving. Some foods may make claims about dietary fiber right on the front of the package. These claims can only be used if the food meets strict FDA definitions. Here are definitions for some label lingo concerning fiber:

- **"Good Source of Fiber":** 3 to less than 5 grams of fiber.
- **"Contains Fiber" or "Provides Fiber":** 10 to 19 percent of the daily value for fiber.
- **"High Fiber," "Rich in Fiber," or "Excellent Source of Fiber":** 5 grams or more fiber (20 percent or more of the daily value for fiber).

These values refer to standard serving sizes. Some fiber claims have higher nutrient levels for main dish products and meal products, such as frozen entrées and/or dinners.

Table 8-1   Foods That Contain Fiber

Food	Serving Size	Fiber (grams)	Food	Serving Size	Fiber (grams)
Fruit			**Beans/lentils, cooked** (continued)		
Apple with skin	1 medium	3	Lentils	½ cup	4
Banana	1 medium	2	Navy beans	½ cup	4
Blueberries	½ cup	2	White beans	½ cup	4.5
Figs, dried	2	4	**Breads and Grains**		
Orange	1 medium	3	Brown rice, cooked	½ cup	2
Orange juice	¾ cup	<1	Pumpernickel bread	1 slice	3
Pear with skin	1 medium	4	Wheat bran	1 tablespoon	2
Strawberries	1 cup	4	Whole-wheat bread	1 slice	2
Vegetables			**Cereals**		
Broccoli, cooked	½ cup	2	100 percent bran	⅓ cup	8
Brussels sprouts, cooked	½ cup	3	Bran flakes	¾ cup	5
Carrots, raw	1 medium	2	Oatmeal, cooked	¾ cup	3
Potato, baked with skin	1 medium	4	Raisin bran	¾ cup	5
Spinach, cooked	½ cup	2	**Snack Foods**		
Tomato, raw	1 medium	2	Peanuts, dry roasted	¼ cup	3
Beans/lentils, cooked			Popcorn, air popped	1 cup	1
Baked beans	½ cup	3	Sunflower seeds	¼ cup	2
Kidney beans	½ cup	3			

Water: A Nutrient for Life

Water is one of the most important and one of the most overlooked nutrients. You can survive for almost six weeks without food, but you cannot survive more than one week without water. Water is one of the most abundant substances in your body and is the nutrient your body needs in the greatest amounts. Almost 55 to 75 percent of an adult's body weight is water. Water is present in every part of your body: it comprises 83 percent of blood, 73 percent of muscle, 25 percent of body fat, and even 22 percent of bones. Since muscle holds more water than body fat, the more muscular you are, the more body water you have and the more water you need.

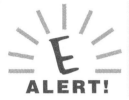

ALERT!

Water is so important to the body that losing just 10 percent of your body weight from dehydration or some other type of water loss can be very dangerous to your health. Losing 20 percent can even be life threatening.

Drinking Water for Health

What better choice for a beverage: water has no calories, is naturally low in sodium, has no fat or cholesterol, has no caffeine, and tastes great! Besides those great qualities, water has a vital role in almost every major function in the body. It does a lot more than just quench your thirst. Water helps to regulate body temperature through perspiration. It transports nutrients and oxygen through the body, carries waste products away from the body cells, cushions joints, and protects body organs. Water is the solution in which all other nutrients are dissolved. It serves as a shock absorber inside the eyes and spinal cord. This amazing nutrient also moistens body tissues in your eyes, mouth, and nose. Water is vital to the digestive process: some of the water in your body comes from the breakdown or metabolism of carbohydrates, proteins, and fats. Water also helps soften the stool to prevent constipation.

How Much We Need

The body has no provision to store water. Therefore, the amount of water lost each day must be continually replaced to maintain good health and proper body function. On average, we lose about 10 cups of water each day just through perspiration, breathing, urination, and bowel movements. This does not include hot days or exercise when you perspire even more. The average adult needs 8 to 12 cups of water each day. To avoid dehydration, the body needs an ongoing supply of water throughout the day. By the time you feel thirsty, you can already be on your way to becoming dehydrated. Losing just 1 to 2 pounds of your body's weight can make you begin to feel thirsty. Your body may require more water in some situations, such as the following:

- Exposure to extreme climates, such as very hot or very cold.
- Performing strenuous work or exercise.
- Eating a high-fiber diet.
- Pregnancy or breastfeeding.
- Prolonged exposure to heated or recirculated air, such as on an airplane.
- Being sick with fever, diarrhea, or vomiting.

Your water needs also increase with both activity level and body weight. The best thing to do is to start with at least 8 cups of water per day and increase it from there as needed. In healthy people, the kidneys simply eliminate any excess water.

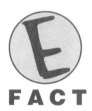

FACT

Dehydration occurs when the body loses excess body water or when the body doesn't get enough water. Symptoms of dehydration can be mild, such as dry skin, fatigue, or loss of endurance and strength. Or they can be far more serious, ranging from poor concentration and headaches to blurred vision and lack of neuromuscular control.

Proper Hydration

When we stay properly hydrated, we have more energy, an improved sense of well-being, greater endurance and stamina during physical activity, and improved digestion and elimination. One of the most common causes of constipation is not being properly hydrated. Good hydration may also help to reduce overeating: many times people grab something to eat when they are not actually hungry but thirsty. To be sure you are properly hydrated, check your urine to make sure it is clear (meaning diluted) rather than a darker yellow.

What to Drink

Plain simple water is the most available and convenient beverage around. If you are trying to avoid extra calories, water is a great choice. The calories in beverages such as soft drinks and alcohol can really add up. Beverages that contain caffeine or alcohol are also not your best choice because they act as diuretics, causing the body to lose needed water through increased urination. It is best to drink these types of beverages in moderation.

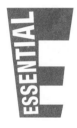

Sparkling water is water with a fizz. This product either has carbon dioxide added or the water is naturally carbonated. By regulation, if carbon dioxide is added, it cannot be any more than its naturally carbonated level would be. If beverages contain sugar, they cannot be considered a water product and must be labeled as a soft drink.

The government strictly regulates both tap water and bottled water. Many people choose bottled water because it does not contain chlorine, which can add a chemical taste to water. Check labels carefully because some clear bottled beverages such as seltzer water or flavored waters can contain sugar and sodium.

Sports drinks contain carbohydrates, which can help supply energy or fuel to muscles during endurance sports. The carbohydrates in sports drinks are usually simple sugars that are absorbed quickly for fast energy. Most sports drinks contain 5 to 8 percent sugar, whereas soft drinks are a much more concentrated source. Carbonated, sugary drinks take longer to be absorbed into the body, which can lead to cramps, diarrhea, or nausea. Most sports drinks also contain electrolytes, such as sodium and potassium, that are lost when athletes perspire heavily. For the average exerciser, sports drinks are not necessary. Water will do just fine. You may benefit from the loaded stuff if you are exercising longer than an hour or are exercising in extremely hot weather.

Tips for Increasing Your Water Intake

It doesn't matter how you do it. It is just important to drink water! Like everything else, drinking water needs to be part of your lifestyle and needs to become an automatic habit. There are all kinds of creative ways you can get yourself to drink your eight glasses of water daily. Try some of these tips:

- Don't put it off; there is nothing like the present. Make a commitment today to start drinking water on a regular basis.
- Start out with a moderate goal and work your way up. Start a water diary on a calendar so you can keep track of your current intake and your progress.
- At work or at home, get in the habit of taking water breaks instead of coffee breaks.
- Keep a bottle of water at your desk, on your counter at home, or in your car when traveling so you continually have it available to sip throughout the day.
- Have a glass of water before and with meals and snacks. Besides helping you to get some water in, it can help take the edge off of your appetite.
- Use a straw to drink your water. Believe it or not, using a straw can help you drink faster and make a glass of water not seem so big.
- Drink water instead of snacking while watching television or reading a book.
- Use a larger cup or water bottle. That way, once you finish it, you are much closer to drinking all of your water for the day. It also helps 64 ounces not seem like so much.
- Keep a 2-quart container of water in the refrigerator, and try emptying it by the time your day is done. This also gives you a constant supply of good cold water.
- Keep a bottle of water with you when you exercise or when you are doing physical activity such as mowing the lawn or cleaning the house.
- Save the money you would have spent on soda or other beverages when drinking water instead. The savings can add up to a lot by the end of the year!
- Substitute sparkling water for alcoholic drinks at social gatherings.

Water and Exercise

When we exercise, we make our internal temperatures rise. Our body cools itself by sweating or perspiring. Sweating causes the body to lose water, so it is important to drink even more water to keep the body cool and to replace lost fluids. The harder and longer your workout, the greater your sweat loss and the more fluid you need to replace.

It is important to drink water before, during, and after you exercise. To prevent dehydration during exercise, experts recommend the following:

- Drinking 2 cups or 16 ounces of fluid, preferably water, two hours prior to exercise.
- Drinking 2 cups of fluid just prior to or up to fifteen minutes before exercise.
- Drinking ½ cup of fluid every fifteen minutes during activity.
- Drinking 2 cups of fluid for every pound lost during your activity.

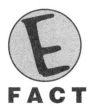

FACT

People who are very fit actually sweat more and start sweating at a lower body temperature. This is because the function of sweating is to cool the body; a physically fit body cools itself more efficiently than one that is unfit.

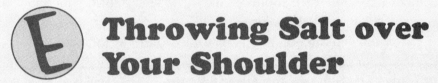

Chapter 9

Throwing Salt over Your Shoulder

Throughout history, salt has had economic as well as symbolic value. In the past it was used heavily for preserving certain foods. Europeans threw salt over their left shoulders to help ward off evil. We do need sodium in our diets every day, but too much sodium leads to adverse health effects.

Salt vs. Sodium

The terms "salt" and "sodium" are often used interchangeably, yet they are two different things. Most problems that come from eating too much salt are really caused by the part of salt called "sodium." Salt, or table salt, is actually the more common name for "sodium chloride." Sodium chloride is 40 percent sodium and 60 percent chloride, meaning table salt is actually 40 percent sodium.

Sodium is a mineral that is naturally found in foods. It is also added to foods for various reasons. It is even present naturally in drinking water, though you don't have to worry about that unless you are on a very low sodium diet. Convenience and/or processed foods contain the most sodium in the form of salt and food additives. Almost three-quarters of the sodium that Americans consume comes from processed and prepared foods.

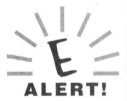

ALERT!

Soft water can be a significant source of sodium, which can be problematic for people on sodium-restricted diets. If you use water softener in your home, avoid excess sodium in your drinking water by buying low-sodium bottled water or installing a separate faucet in the kitchen that dispenses unsoftened water.

Sodium and Your Health

Even though you often hear bad press about sodium, it is important to remember that this mineral is essential to life. Sodium is an electrolyte, along with chloride and potassium, and the body needs it in certain amounts to help maintain fluid balance. Sodium helps control the flow of fluids into and out of each cell. By regulating fluids, electrolytes such as sodium aid the absorption of nutrients across cell membranes and maintain your body's acid/base balance. Sodium also assists in regulating blood pressure, sparking nerve impulses, and helping muscles including the heart to relax. Sodium also helps the body process and digest proteins and carbohydrates.

Sodium Recommendations

Though there is no Recommended Dietary Allowance (RDA), the American Heart Association recommends that healthy American adults eat no more than 2,400 mg of sodium per day. The National Academy of Sciences has established a minimum level of at least 500 mg to help keep the body running properly. The following list illustrates just how much sodium is in certain amounts of table salt:

- ¼ teaspoon salt = 500 mg sodium
- ½ teaspoon salt = 1,000 mg sodium
- ¾ teaspoon salt = 1,500 mg sodium
- 1 teaspoon salt = 2,000 mg sodium

Most Americans consume far more than the recommended levels. The average sodium intake in the United States is between 4,000 and 6,000 mg per day. Salt is a key ingredient in many foods, making it very easy to get enough sodium by consuming an average diet without having to get extra from the saltshaker. Moderation is the key to sodium intake.

Too Much Sodium

In healthy people, the kidneys help regulate the sodium level in the body. Sodium levels usually don't become too high because most excess sodium is excreted from the body in urine and through perspiration. For example, when you eat foods that are high in salt, you probably urinate more frequently because your body is trying to rid itself of the extra sodium. Even though your sodium intake may vary from day to day, your body is very efficient at maintaining a proper balance.

Everyone has felt the effects of swollen fingers or feeling a bit bloated. It is common to feel these effects after eating very salty foods. This is because the body requires a certain balance of sodium and water. If you eat extra sodium, the body needs extra water in the cells, which usually results in water retention. Drinking extra fluids, especially water, helps balance the sodium-water concentration and relieve the fluid retention. The reason you usually are thirstier after eating salty foods is that salt triggers your thirst response, telling your body you need more water to balance it out.

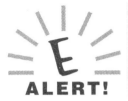

ALERT!

Women who are pregnant should not decrease their sodium intake to minimize water retention or swelling without their doctor's consent. During pregnancy the body's need for sodium actually increases.

The Scoop on Sodium

When kidneys don't work properly because of problems like kidney disease, they cannot rid the body of excess sodium, causing edema, or swelling in legs and feet. Though fairly rare, individuals can develop sodium deficiency, which is called "hyponatremia." This deficiency can be the result of profuse sweating, prolonged vomiting or diarrhea, diuretics or water pills, or kidney disease. Symptoms may include dizziness, muscle cramps, muscle weakness, headaches, and nausea.

Sodium's Link to High Blood Pressure

High blood pressure, or hypertension, is a major risk factor for heart disease, stroke, and kidney disease. As your heart beats, blood flows from the heart out to the blood vessels. This flow creates pressure against the blood vessel walls. Your blood pressure reading is a measure of this pressure. When that reading goes above a certain point, it is called high blood pressure. High blood pressure can occur when too much pressure is placed on the walls of the arteries, when there is an increase in blood volume, or when the blood vessels constrict or narrow. High blood pressure makes the heart work harder, and over time it can damage the artery walls.

High blood pressure is not particular. It can strike anyone, regardless of race, age, or gender. According to a National Heart, Lung, and Blood Institute estimate, one in every four Americans—or nearly 50 million people—has high blood pressure. Hypertension is especially dangerous because it often has no warning signs or symptoms. Of those people with high blood pressure, almost 32 percent don't even know that they have it. Fortunately, it is easy to monitor your blood pressure by having it checked regularly. The cause of 90 to 95 percent of the cases of high blood pressure isn't known; however, high blood pressure is easily detected and usually controllable.

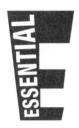

Blood pressure is recorded as two numbers—the systolic pressure (as the heart beats) over the diastolic pressure (as the heart relaxes between beats). The measurement is written one above the other, with the systolic number on top and the diastolic number on the bottom. For example, a blood pressure measurement of 120/80 mm Hg (millimeters of mercury) is expressed verbally as "120 over 80."

Table 9-1	American Heart Association Recommendations on Blood Pressure Readings			
Blood Pressure (mm Hg)	**Optimal**	**Normal**	**High Normal**	**Hypertension**
Systolic (top number)	less than 120	less than 130	130–139	140 or higher
Diastolic (bottom number)	less than 80	less than 85	85–89	90 or higher

Blood Pressure, Sodium, and Your Kidneys

The regulation of blood pressure is closely linked to the kidneys' ability to excrete enough sodium to maintain normal sodium balance, extracellular fluid volume, and blood volume. In normal healthy people, the body adjusts to a higher intake of sodium. The body excretes more sodium without raising arterial pressure. However, many outside influences, as well as kidney problems, can lead to the body's reduced capability to excrete sodium. With a normal or higher salt intake, if the kidneys cannot excrete sodium, the result is a chronic increase in extracellular fluid and blood volume. These conditions lead to high blood pressure.

Are You Sodium Sensitive?

Most people are not affected by excess sodium because the excess is excreted in the urine, but 30 percent of Americans have blood pressure that is sensitive to sodium. Too much sodium in these people can cause high blood pressure. These people cannot efficiently excrete sodium, which means it hangs around, drawing in water, and increasing blood volume. The increase in blood volume can then stimulate the vessels to constrict, creating an increase in pressure or blood pressure.

Some people who do not have high blood pressure or who have sodium-sensitive blood pressure may reduce their risk by eating a diet with less sodium.

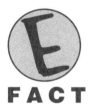

There is no way to predict whether a person will develop high blood pressure or if he or she would benefit from reducing sodium intake. Therefore, the best advice for most people is to just eat less salt. Most people already consume much more than they need, and a reduction will most likely benefit those people whose blood pressure may be sodium sensitive.

A high-sodium diet alone does not cause high blood pressure. It is a combination of certain risk factors. Some of these factors cannot be controlled, such as age (as you get older your risk increases), race (African-Americans tend to have high blood pressure more often than other races), and a family history of high blood pressure. Other risk factors can be controlled, such as sodium consumption, obesity, physical activity, smoking, and alcohol consumption.

Sodium in Your Diet

Sodium in your diet can come from both natural and added sodium sources. The amount of sodium found naturally in food is not high enough for concern. Most of the sodium you eat comes from salt added during food processing or during preparation in a restaurant or at home.

Sodium in food is used as a preservative and stabilizer as well as for flavor. High amounts of salt, or sodium chloride, are found in processed meats such as bacon, sausage, hot dogs, and ham; in canned soups and vegetables; in many frozen foods; and in fast foods. Sodium is also found in pickles, olives, nuts, cereals, baked goods, and snack foods like potato chips. Most restaurant food is also high in sodium. Foods described with the words "broth," "cured," "corned," "pickled," and "smoked" usually contain sodium. It is important to look for certain words on packaged food to clue you in that the product contains sodium. Sodium-containing food additives include the following:

- Brine
- Disodium phosphate
- Monosodium glutamate (MSG)
- Sodium nitrite
- Sodium sulfite
- Baking soda, or sodium bicarbonate
- Baking powder
- Sodium chloride (table salt)
- Soy sauce

- Teriyaki sauce
- Sodium benzoate
- Sodium caseinate
- Sodium citrate
- Sodium nitrate
- Sodium propionate
- Sodium sulfite
- Worcestershire sauce

Certain types of foods contain a lot of sodium. When we combine these foods with the amount of salt we typically sprinkle on food, our sodium intake can add up quickly. It is essential to be aware of foods that are higher and/or lower in sodium to help you moderate your sodium intake.

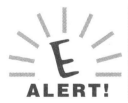

ALERT!

Many medications contain sodium, such as antacids, headache remedies, laxatives, and sedatives. If you are on a sodium-restricted diet, talk to your doctor and/or pharmacist about the sodium content of any medications you are taking.

Table 9-2   Sodium Content of Foods

Type of Food	Sodium Content (mg)
Meat, Poultry, Fish, and Shellfish	
Fresh meat (beef, pork, lamb, veal), poultry, finfish (cooked); 3 ounces	>90
Clams (steamed); 3 ounces	95
Tuna (canned); 3 ounces	300
Chicken hot dog; 1	755
Lean ham; 3 ounces	1,025
Dairy Products	
Skim or 1 percent milk; 1 cup	125
Buttermilk (salt added); 1 cup	260
Yogurt, low-fat or nonfat, fruited; 8 ounces	120–150
Yogurt, low-fat or nonfat, plain; 8 ounces	160–175
Cheese, low-fat; 1 ounce	150
Cheese, low-fat and low sodium; 1 ounce	**Read the label**
Cottage cheese, low-fat; ½ cup	460
Eggs	
Egg white; 1	55
Egg substitute; ¼ cup = 1 egg	80–120
Fats and Oils	
Oil; 1 tablespoon	0
Unsalted tub margarine; 1 teaspoon	>5
Salted tub margarine; 1 teaspoon	45
Prepared salad dressings, low calorie; 2 tablespoons	50–310
Imitation mayonnaise, nonfat; 1 tablespoon	110

Type of Food	Sodium Content (mg)
Fruits	
Fruits (fresh, frozen, canned); ½ cup	>10
Vegetables	
Fresh or frozen vegetables (cooked without salt); ½ cup	>70
Canned vegetables; ½ cup	170
Tomato juice (canned); ¾ cup	660
Breads, Cereals, Rice, Pasta, and Dry Peas and Beans	
Corn tortilla; 1	40
Bread; 1 slice	110–175
Melba toast; 3 rectangles	120
English muffin; ½	130
Bagel; ½	190
Rice, plain brown or white; 1 cup	5
Rice, boxed convenience rice; 1 cup	1,600
Cracker, saltine type; 5 squares	195
Ready-to-Eat Cereal	
Shredded Wheat; ¾ cup	>5
Puffed wheat and rice; 1½ to 1⅔ cups	>5
Granola type; ½ cup	5–25
Ring and nugget cereals; 1 cup	170–310
Flaked cereals; ⅔ to 1 cup	170–360

continued on facing page

Table 9-2 Sodium Content of Foods *(continued)*

Type of Food	Sodium Content (mg)
Cooked cereal	
Cooked cereal (unsalted); 1/2 cup	>5
Instant cooked cereal; 3/4 cup	180
Rice and pasta (unsalted); 1/2 cup	>10
Peanut butter; 2 tablespoons	150
Peanut butter (unsalted); 2 tablespoons	>5
Dry beans, plain, canned (salted); 1/2 cup	350–590
Dry beans, home cooked (unsalted, canned); 1/2 cup	>5
Snacks	
Popcorn and nuts (unsalted); 1 ounce	>10
Popcorn and nuts (salted); 1 ounce	170–250
Jellybeans; 10 large	5
Hard candy; 1 ounce	10
Vanilla wafers; 1	10
Fig bar cookies; 1	55
Angel food cake; 1/12 of a 9-inch cake	210
Ice pop; 1	10
Frozen nonfat or low-fat yogurt; 1/2 cup	40–55
Ice milk; 1/2 cup	55–60

Type of Food	Sodium Content (mg)
Condiments	
Mustard, chili sauce, hot sauce; 1 teaspoon	35–65
Ketchup, steak sauce; 1 teaspoon	100–230
Salt; 1/6 teaspoon	390
Pickles; 1 medium dill	835
Soy sauce; 1 tablespoon	1,030
Soy sauce, lower sodium; 1 tablespoon	600
Worcestershire sauce; 1 tablespoon	234
Convenience Foods	
Canned and dehydrated soups; 1 cup	600–1,300
Canned and dehydrated soups, lower-sodium version; 1 cup	50
Chicken broth; 1 cup	1,005
Chicken broth, lower-sodium version; 1 cup	70
Canned and frozen main dishes; 8 ounces	500–1,570
Canned and frozen main dishes, lower-sodium versions; 8 ounces	(Read the label)

Decreasing Your Sodium Intake

It is important to remember that the bottom line is to reduce, not eliminate, higher-sodium foods from your diet. Reducing the salt in your diet does not have to mean giving up the pleasure of great-tasting foods. Learning to use less sodium takes time and flexibility. It needs to become a lifestyle change. Here are some tips for cutting sodium in your diet to an advised amount:

- Begin to gradually decrease salt or sodium intake, especially if you are accustomed to salty tastes.
- Eat lots of fresh fruits and vegetables.
- Choose lower-sodium foods by learning to read food labels.
- Use herbs and spices to season foods instead of salt.
- Taste foods first before adding salt.
- Cook foods such as noodles, rice, and hot cereals without adding salt.
- Use less salt when preparing your favorite recipes.
- Eat slightly salted or unsalted crackers, pretzels, nuts, and other usually salted food.
- Leave the saltshaker off the table during meals.
- Choose fresh foods over processed, canned, and prepared foods (frozen vegetables are usually lower in sodium) more often.
- Look for labels that say "low sodium." These foods contain 140 mg or less of sodium per serving.
- If you eat frozen convenience foods often, look for products with less than 800 mg sodium per serving.
- Go easy on condiments such as ketchup, soy sauce, teriyaki sauce, mustard, pickles, and olives.

Conquer Your Craving for Salt

Ever wonder just why you love salty foods? Well, people with a strong taste for salty foods have actually acquired that taste. The preference usually starts in childhood and has a lot to do with the foods you ate growing up. It is a learned behavior that can be unlearned. When people begin to lower salt and sodium in the diet, their desire for salty foods actually begins to decrease. Food can still have plenty of flavors even with less salt.

Salt Substitute Solutions

Salt substitutes are available on the market today as a way to moderate your sodium intake. Salt substitutes are not for everyone, though. Substitutes are usually made of potassium chloride instead of sodium chloride. For some people, such as those with kidney problems, large amounts of potassium can be harmful because these people are not able to excrete excess potassium. Even the "lite" salt products on the market are half salt (sodium chloride) and half salt substitute (potassium chloride). People trying to decrease sodium intake should check with their physicians before using salt substitutes or lite salt products, especially if already under a doctor's care. Rather than salt substitutes, try blends of herbs and spices to flavor foods. You can also try the lower-salt vegetable seasoning shakers that are now on the market.

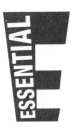

To moderate salt intake without using salt substitutes, try this blend of herbs and spices as an alternative: ½ teaspoon of cayenne pepper, 1 tablespoon of garlic powder, and 1 teaspoon each of ground basil, ground marjoram, ground thyme, parsley, savory, mace, onion powder, black pepper, and sage. Combine all the seasonings in a salt shaker with large holes. Use the shaker in cooking or at the table to season food to taste.

Dining Out

When you eat out, it is more difficult to be aware of the sodium content of the food you are eating. However, you can take some steps to dramatically reduce the sodium content of your restaurant meal and still enjoy it, such as the following:

• Leave the saltshaker off the table or move it to another table. Use pepper, lemon juice, or request herbs and spices as an alternative.

- Go easy on condiments such as ketchup, mustard, salad dressing, and sauces.
- Ask your server questions about how food is prepared, and don't be afraid to ask that your food be prepared without salt.
- Recognize certain words that may indicate that the food is higher in sodium, such as smoked, pickled, marinated, teriyaki, soy sauce, broth, or au jus.
- Try nibbling on fresh veggies instead of salty snacks such as tortilla chips.
- Order foods that are not served with special sauces or gravies. Often these toppings can add a ton of extra sodium to your meal.
- Watch out for entrées with large amounts of cheese.
- If making a salad at the salad bar, beware of higher-sodium toppings such as cheese, olives, dressings, croutons, and canned vegetables.

Sodium Label Lingo

Using the food label or nutrition claims on the front of a packaged food can clue you in to how much sodium may be in the product. The food label lists sodium content in milligrams per serving. The place to begin is the "Percent Daily Value" column under the Nutrition Facts Panel. The numbers in this column show whether a food is high or low in a specific nutrient. Though important for everyone, the Percent Daily Value for sodium is especially important for people who have high blood pressure or are on a low-sodium diet. If the Percent Daily Value for sodium is 5 or less, the food is considered low in that nutrient. The goal should be to select, as much as possible, foods that have a value of 5 or less. The goal for the full day's diet should be to select foods that together add up to no more than 100 percent of the daily value for sodium, which is 2,400 mg.

If you see a nutritional claim including the words "sodium" or "salt" on a food package, it is important to understand what that claim means. Here's a description of some common claims:

- **Sodium free or salt free:** less than 5 mg per serving.
- **Very low sodium:** 35 mg or less per serving or, if the serving is 30 g or less or 2 tablespoons or less, 35 mg or less per 50 g of the food.
- **Low sodium:** 140 mg or less per serving or, if the serving is 30 g or less or 2 tablespoons or less, 140 mg or less per 50 g of the food.
- **Light in sodium:** at least 50 percent less sodium per serving than the average reference amount for same food with no sodium reduction; restricted to foods with more than 40 calories per serving or more than 3 grams fat per serving.
- **Reduced or less sodium:** at least 25 percent less (as compared with a standard serving size of the traditional food) sodium per serving.
- **Unsalted, without added salt, no salt added:** no salt added during processing; does not mean sodium free.

The FDA and USDA state that a food that has the claim "healthy" cannot exceed 360 mg of sodium per reference amount or serving size. Foods that are meals must not exceed 480 mg per reference amount to use the claim "healthy."

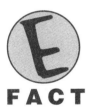

FACT

If a food is not "sodium free," the statement "not a sodium-free food" or "not for control of sodium in the diet" must appear on the same panel as the Nutrition Facts Panel.

Chapter 10

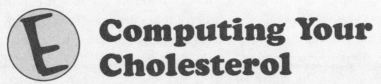 Computing Your Cholesterol

Cholesterol can be a confusing topic. There are good and bad cholesterol; there are blood and dietary cholesterol. What does it all mean? It is important to learn what cholesterol is, how it can affect your health, and how to manage your dietary intake and blood cholesterol levels.

What Is Cholesterol?

Cholesterol is a waxy, fatlike substance found in tissue and in the blood. Our bodies manufacture about 80 percent of our cholesterol supply, and we get the rest by eating certain foods, especially saturated fats. Cholesterol that is found in food is called dietary cholesterol, and the type found in your bloodstream is referred to as blood or serum cholesterol. Many factors affect blood cholesterol. The cholesterol that circulates in your body comes from both the cholesterol your body produces and from the foods you eat.

Even though you often see cholesterol listed among dietary fat, cholesterol is not the same as fat.

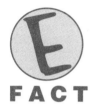

FACT

When triggered by sunlight, cholesterol in your skin has the ability to convert to vitamin D, which is an essential vitamin that is needed for building bone.

Cholesterol differs from fat in that it possesses a different type of structure and performs separate functions in the body. Cholesterol also differs from fat in that it is not broken down in the body and therefore does not provide energy and calories. Eating too much fat can cause you to gain weight, while cholesterol cannot.

Cholesterol is essential for maintaining healthy cell function and is required by the body to insulate nerves, create cell membranes, and produce certain hormones such as estrogen and testosterone. It is part of every body cell and is also a component of bile, which helps the body to digest and absorb needed fat. In moderation, cholesterol is essential to many bodily functions. However, our body makes plenty of cholesterol, and most dietary cholesterol we consume is considered to be excess.

The Good and the Bad

There are different types of blood cholesterol. Cholesterol in food is neither good nor bad. In food, it's all the same. The cholesterol that is referred to as "good" (HDL) and "bad" (LDL) refers only to the cholesterol found in your bloodstream. However, your food choices can directly influence your LDL-cholesterol levels.

In the body, cholesterol travels through the bloodstream by attaching to protein groups called lipoproteins. The two main lipoproteins are low-density lipoproteins (LDLs) and high-density lipoproteins (HDLs).

HDL Cholesterol

The term "good cholesterol" refers to HDL or high-density lipoproteins. HDL carries about one-third to one-fourth of blood cholesterol. HDL cholesterol is known as the good cholesterol because a high level of HDL cholesterol may help to protect against heart disease. The function of HDL is to gather cholesterol from every part of the body and carry it back to the liver for disposal. HDL is also referred to as "good" because some experts believe that it helps to remove excess cholesterol from plaque, a thick, hard deposit that can clog major arteries. An HDL cholesterol level of less than 40 mg/dL is considered too low. A low HDL level can put you at a higher risk for heart disease. Many factors can contribute to a lower HDL-cholesterol level. If you have low HDL cholesterol, you can help raise it by doing the following:

- Not smoking
- Losing weight (or maintaining a healthy weight)
- Being physically active for at least thirty to sixty minutes per day on most days of the week

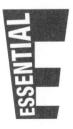

Your ratio of HDL cholesterol to total cholesterol is also an important factor. For example, if you have a total cholesterol of 200 and an HDL level of 50, the ratio would be 4:1. Your goal should be to keep the ratio below 5:1. The optimum ratio is 3.5:1, according to the American Heart Association.

LDL Cholesterol

LDL, or low-density lipoproteins, is called "bad cholesterol." High levels of LDL are associated with an increased risk for heart disease, heart attack, and stroke. Therefore a lower level of LDL cholesterol is linked to a decreased risk of heart disease. The function of LDL is to carry cholesterol from the liver to other tissues.

When there is too much LDL cholesterol circulating in the bloodstream, it can slowly build up on the walls of the arteries that supply blood to the heart and brain. This can contribute to the formation of plaque that can clog those major arteries. This health condition is known as atherosclerosis. If a clot forms where there is already a plaque formation, the blood flow can be blocked completely to part of the heart muscle, which can ultimately cause a heart attack. If a clot forms and blocks the blood flow to the brain, a stroke can result.

Your LDL cholesterol can be categorized into one of the following:

- **Desirable:** less than 130 mg/dL
- **Borderline high risk:** 130–159 mg/dL
- **High risk:** 160 mg/dL or higher

The key point to remember is this: the lower your LDL cholesterol, the lower your risk. The first step your doctor will probably take is to prescribe a diet low in saturated fat and cholesterol, along with regular exercise and weight loss if you are overweight. If you are not successful in lowering your cholesterol through these lifestyle changes, your doctor may then prescribe a prescription medication.

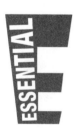

High cholesterol can be a genetic problem. In other words, it may run in your family, giving you a genetic predisposition that causes your body to produce higher amounts of cholesterol. For these people, lifestyle changes probably will not help lower cholesterol levels, and they will need the assistance of cholesterol-lowering medications.

Check Your Blood Cholesterol

It is important to have your blood cholesterol checked regularly because symptoms of high cholesterol are not always obvious. The American Heart Association recommends that all adults aged twenty or older have a fasting lipid profile (total cholesterol, LDL cholesterol, HDL cholesterol, and triglyceride) once every five years.

Cholesterol is measured through blood analysis and is best tested when the person fasts for at least twelve hours prior. The sample is analyzed for total cholesterol and, if the need exists, for LDLs and HDLs. Cholesterol is measured in milligrams per deciliter (mg/dL).

Triglycerides

Triglycerides don't get as much attention as cholesterol, but they are also linked to heart disease. If you have several risk factors for heart disease, your doctor will probably check your triglyceride levels along with your cholesterol. Triglycerides are the main form of fat in foods and in the blood. Your triglyceride level will fall into one of these categories:

- **Normal:** less than 150 mg/dL
- **Borderline to high:** 150–199 mg/dL
- **High:** 200–499 mg/dL
- **Very high:** greater than 500 mg/dL

Because of their roles in metabolism, triglyceride levels are inversely related to HDL-cholesterol levels. When a person has a high triglyceride level, the HDL-cholesterol levels are usually low.

Total Cholesterol Levels

It is important to ask your doctor for a total lipoprotein profile so that you are aware of not only your total cholesterol but of each component of your cholesterol. You may have a total cholesterol level that is desirable, but that doesn't mean your HDL and LDL levels are in line. Your total cholesterol level will fall into one of three categories:

- **Desirable:** less than 200 mg/dL
- **Borderline high risk:** 200–239 mg/dL
- **High risk:** 240 mg/dL and over

If you fall in the desirable range, your risk for heart attack is relatively low. However, it is still smart to get plenty of physical activity and to follow a healthy diet, low in cholesterol and saturated fat, to maintain a healthy weight.

If you fall within the borderline high-risk range, you have at least twice the risk of a heart attack compared with someone who in the desirable range. If you are in this range, your HDL is less than 40 mg/dL, and you don't have other risk factors for heart disease, you should have your total cholesterol and HDL rechecked in one to two years. You should also lower your intake of foods high in saturated fat and cholesterol to help reduce your cholesterol level to below 200. Your doctor may order another blood test to measure your LDL cholesterol. Even if your total cholesterol puts you in the borderline high-risk range, you may not be at high risk for a heart attack. Some people, such as women before menopause, and young, active men with no other risk factors, can have high HDL-cholesterol and desirable LDL levels, so it is best to ask your doctor to interpret your results. Everyone's case is different.

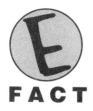

FACT

The American Heart Association now encourages Americans to think of their blood cholesterol as a vital sign similar to blood pressure for measuring heart health.

If your total cholesterol level is 240 or more, you are definitely at high risk. Your risk of heart attack and, indirectly, of stroke are greater. If you fall in this category, you should ask your doctor for advice. About 20 percent of the U.S. population has what is considered high blood cholesterol levels.

The bottom line is that the less LDL you have, and the more HDL you have, the lower your risk for heart disease. When it comes to trying to lower your LDL, your food choices are key.

It is essential to follow your physician's advice after you have had your cholesterol tested.

If you have a cholesterol reading over 240 mg/dL or you have risk factors such as heart disease along with cholesterol readings over 200 mg/dL, your doctor will probably prescribe a cholesterol-lowering medication in combination with a healthy low-fat diet and exercise. There are several different types of these medications on the market today, and your doctor may even prescribe more than one. Your doctor should periodically test your blood cholesterol levels to check on your progress. As with any type of medication that your doctor prescribes, it is essential to follow the recommended dosage and schedule requirements to experience results.

Lowering Your Cholesterol Levels

A combination of a diet low in saturated fat and cholesterol, regular physical activity, and a healthy weight can have many positive effects on your health, including decreasing your risk for heart disease. These elements can help you lower your total cholesterol as well as raise your HDL, lower your LDL, and lower your triglycerides. It is important to focus on your cholesterol intake as well as your saturated fat intake, which often occur together in foods. Cholesterol and most saturated fat come *only* from animal foods. Even though some foods of plant origin are high in fat or saturated fat, all plant foods are cholesterol free. Nuts, for example, are high in fat—mostly unsaturated fat—but are cholesterol free.

A Heart-Healthy Diet

In order to keep your LDL and your risk for heart disease low, it is important to start with a heart-healthy diet. We get cholesterol in two ways. The body, mainly the liver, produces varying amounts of cholesterol each day. Cholesterol also comes directly from animal foods such as egg yolks, meat, poultry, fish, seafood, and whole-milk dairy products.

Typically our body makes all the cholesterol it needs, so we don't need to consume it. Saturated fat is actually the chief culprit in raising blood cholesterol levels. In fact, saturated fat raises your LDL-cholesterol level more than anything else in the diet. *Trans* fats also raise blood cholesterol as well as dietary cholesterol itself.

The American Heart Association recommends "that you limit your average daily cholesterol intake to less than 300 mg. If you have heart disease, limit your daily intake to less than 200 mg. Still, everyone should remember that by keeping their dietary intake of saturated fats low, they can significantly lower their dietary cholesterol intake. Foods high in saturated fat generally contain substantial amounts of dietary cholesterol."

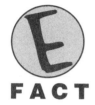

FACT

In the United States, the average dietary cholesterol intake for men is about 337 mg and for women is about 217 mg per day.

A heart-healthy diet consists of the following:

- Consuming 8–10 percent of the day's total calories from saturated fat.
- Consuming 30 percent or less of the day's total calories from fat.
- Consuming less than 300 mg of dietary cholesterol a day.
- Limiting sodium intake to 2,400 mg a day.
- Consuming just enough calories to achieve or maintain a healthy weight and reduce your blood cholesterol level. (Ask your doctor or registered dietitian what is a reasonable calorie level for you.)

To calculate how much 30 percent of your total calories are for total fat and how much 8–10 percent of your total calories are for saturated fat, use the following calculations. These calculations are based on 2,000 calories per day. If you are on a different caloric level, just plug in your calorie level.

To figure out your total fat values for the day, follow these calculations:

1. *To figure total fat calories per day:*
   30 percent (or .30) x 2,000 calories = 600 calories from total fat.
2. *To figure total fat grams per day:*
   600 calories from total fat ÷ 9 calories per gram of fat = 66.66 or 67 grams of total fat per day.

To figure out your total saturated fat values for the day, follow these calculations:

1. *To figure total saturated fat calories per day:*
   10 percent (or .10) x 2,000 calories = 200 calories from saturated fat.
2. *To figure total saturated fat grams per day:*
   200 calories from saturated fat ÷ 9 calories per gram = 22 grams of saturated fat (of the 67 grams of total fat) per day.

Food Culprits

Reducing the amount of total fat, saturated fat, and cholesterol you eat is a very important step in reducing your blood cholesterol levels. Both saturated fat and cholesterol come from animal foods.

To help lower the amount of fat and cholesterol in your daily diet, follow these guidelines:

- Eat at least five servings of fruits and vegetables per day. They are low in fat, and some contain soluble fibers that have a cholesterol-lowering effect.
- Eat lower fat whole-grain products such as breads, cereals, pitas, rice, and pastas.
- Choose lower-fat or nonfat dairy products to help reduce total fat. The needed nutrients in dairy products are the same whether you consume whole-milk or fat-free milk products.
- Consume lean meats, skinless poultry, and fish. Loin and round cuts of meat have less fat. The cholesterol in meat is found both in the fat and the muscle, so trimming fat and buying leaner cuts can help reduce your cholesterol intake.
- Enjoy seafood, prepared in a low-fat way, as your main meal a few times per week.
- Go easy on fats and oils. Instead of using butter or oily sauces at meals, try flavoring with herbs and spices. Buy lower-fat versions of fats such as dressings, mayonnaise, margarine, and cream cheese.

- Make vegetarian meals occasionally. Meals with beans or soy products as the main protein source have several cholesterol-lowering qualities.
- Read food labels to help you keep track of how much fat, saturated fat, and cholesterol you eat in a day.

To specifically reduce saturated fat, follow these additional tips:

- Use liquid vegetable oils instead of solid fats such as shortening and butter. The more soft or liquid a fat is at room temperature, the less saturated fat it has.
- Cut back on your total fat intake to help reduce your saturated fat intake.

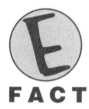

FACT

Even though some shellfish, such as shrimp or lobster, contain higher amounts of cholesterol, it has substantially less total fat and less saturated fat than red meat, so it is a leaner choice.

To specifically help reduce your cholesterol intake, follow these additional guidelines:

- Eat no more than four egg yolks per week. Egg yolks contain about 215 mg from a large egg, but the egg white has *no* cholesterol. Try substituting two egg whites for one whole egg in baked goods or using an egg substitute.
- Limit organ meats such as liver. They are nutritious but also very high in cholesterol.
- Check labels to find foods that are lower in cholesterol.

Cooking Healthy

A healthful eating plan is more than just choosing the right foods to eat. It is also important to prepare and cook foods in a healthy way. Some ways of cooking are better than others when it comes to cutting cholesterol, fat, and calories. At the same time, you want to get as much nutritional value as possible and not give up the taste. All you have to do is just learn some heart-healthy cooking techniques, and you can have a healthy eating plan that tastes good and is good for you. Try these tips:

- Roast with a rack so the meat or poultry doesn't sit in its own fat drippings. Set your oven to 350 degrees to avoid searing. Baste with fat-free liquids like wine, tomato juice, pineapple juice, light teriyaki sauce, or lemon juice.
- Bake in covered cookware with a little extra liquid.
- Braise or stew meats on top of the stove or in the oven. Refrigerate the cooked dish to harden the saturated fat and make it easy to remove the fat before reheating.
- Poach chicken or fish by immersing it in simmering nonfat liquid.
- Grill or broil on a rack so fat drips away from the food.
- Sauté in an open skillet over high heat. Use a nonstick vegetable spray, a small amount of broth or wine, or a small amount of olive oil rubbed on the pan with a paper towel.
- Stir-fry with a small amount of olive oil in a wok or large deep fry pan.
- When you microwave you need no extra fat to cook with. In fact, you can drain food of fat by placing it between two paper towels while it cooks.
- Steam in a basket over simmering water. (Great for vegetables!)

How to Cut the Fat

Most Americans consume, on average, about 34 percent or more of their calories from fat. The health benefits of cutting back are remarkable. There are many ways to trim fat and cholesterol from your diet, but remember: it is not necessary to do them all at the same time. Try a few strategies, and once you have mastered those, try a few more. You can cut the fat and cholesterol in your meals without having to lose any flavor. Start with one of these techniques:

- After browning, put ground meat into a strainer lined with paper towels. Or rinse it. Leave in the pan and rinse with hot water several times.
- To make gravy without fat, blend 1 tablespoon of cornstarch with a

cup of room-temperature broth by shaking them together in a jar. Heat the remainder of the broth, add the blended liquid, and simmer until thick.

- Prepare scrambled eggs or omelets by using only one egg yolk per serving and adding a few extra egg whites to the batch. Or use an egg substitute product instead.
- Remove oils in canned tuna, salmon, or sardines by draining and/or rinsing them in cool water. Even better: buy the varieties canned in water instead of oil.
- Don't overcook vegetables. Lightly steam them instead of boiling them to help keep more of their natural flavor, fiber, and nutrients.
- Mix creamy salad dressing with plain low-fat yogurt.
- Use finely chopped vegetables to stretch ground poultry or meat.
- Use herbs and spices to add flavor to foods.

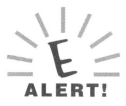

ALERT!

Although it is important to good health to eat a low-fat diet, every diet must contain some fat. Fat is responsible for many essential functions in the body. A completely fat-free diet can be dangerous and is not recommended.

Fiber, Vitamin E, and Garlic

No single food will lower your blood cholesterol. However, foods that are high in soluble fibers may help to lower LDL-cholesterol levels. Studies have shown that foods such as oatmeal that are high in soluble fiber may help to lower LDL cholesterol without lowering HDL cholesterol. Foods high in soluble fibers include oatmeal, oat bran, barley, dry beans or legumes, peas, and some fruits and vegetables. Quick ways to pack fiber into your day include eating from all five food groups; eating fiber-rich grains, such as oatmeal or whole-grain cereals, at breakfast; picking high-fiber snacks such as popcorn, fresh fruit, and fresh vegetables; and "fiberizing" your cooking style by swapping higher fiber ingredients in recipes; and eating at least five servings of fruits and vegetables each day.

Vitamin E is a powerful antioxidant that helps to protect cells from damage caused by substances called free radicals. Research shows that vitamin E may help prevent or delay heart disease by targeting the free radicals that combine with LDL cholesterol in the body. Results of several studies now show that consuming fruits, vegetables, and whole grains that contain antioxidants such as vitamin E may help lower the risk for heart disease. However, it is still unclear whether taking antioxidant supplements in the form of pills has a similar benefit and how much is needed. Foods high in vitamin E include vegetable oils, foods made from vegetable oils such as salad dressing and margarine, nuts, seeds, and wheat germ. Leafy green vegetables provide a smaller amount.

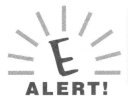

ALERT!

Check with your doctor before taking any type of supplement in amounts that exceed the Recommended Daily Allowance (RDA) or Daily Recommended Intake (DRI).

Garlic has been touted as effective in lowering cholesterol levels. Studies are inconclusive as to whether this is true. Garlic appears to have certain compounds that may help lower cholesterol, but most studies show that the benefit comes from the garlic itself, not a capsule or oil. The effective amount is still in question. Until more is known, get the benefits of garlic by using it when cooking stir-fries, salads, pasta, chicken, rice, or any of your favorite low-fat meals.

Cholesterol-Lowering Margarines

Various margarines on the market today are low in both saturated fats and trans fatty acids. Trans fatty acids are created through the process of hydrogenation. They can increase LDL cholesterol and lower HDL. Many of these margarines are called "spreads" because they are less than 80 percent oil. The more solid a margarine is, the more saturated fat and trans fat they contain. For instance, stick margarine in general contains higher amounts of trans fats than tub margarines. When looking for margarine spreads, keep the following things in mind.

- Look for a margarine spread with no more than 30 percent fat from saturated plus trans fat. Less than 20 percent is even better.
- Pay attention to calories in your spread. Whether a spread has good (unsaturated fats) or bad fat (saturated fats), it is still a lot of calories for a small serving. A "light" spread will have fewer calories, but remember that less fat means more water, so you may not be able to use it for baking or sautéing.
- Consider claims that you see on the package. Look for words such as "trans-free," which means the spread has no more than half a gram of trans fat per serving. But be sure they are not replacing trans fats with saturated fats.

These new margarine spreads are not a magic bullet to lowering cholesterol, but in moderation they can be part of your heart-healthy lifestyle.

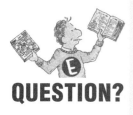

QUESTION?

Can fish oil help lower your cholesterol levels?
The American Heart Association recommends eating fish two times per week. Fatty fish like mackerel, lake trout, herring, sardines, albacore tuna, and salmon are also high in omega-3 fatty acids, which may have health benefits. Fish is a good source of protein without the high saturated fat and cholesterol found in fatty meat products. At this point, the benefits and risks of taking fish oil still need to be defined by further research.

Cholesterol and Fat Label Lingo

The food label or nutrition claims on packaged foods can clue you in to how much fat and cholesterol are in the product. The food label lists fat and saturated fat content in grams per serving and lists cholesterol in milligrams per serving.

A good place to begin is the Percent Daily Value column in the Nutrition Facts Panel. This column shows whether a food is high or low in a specific nutrient. The Percent Daily Value for cholesterol is based on

300 mg. It stays the same, no matter how many calories you consume each day. The Percent Daily value for total fat is based on 65 grams and for saturated fat is based on 20 grams. These numbers are calculated using a 2,000-calorie diet. Your total amount of fat and saturated fat may differ slightly depending on how many calories you eat per day. You can calculate these numbers using the formulas in the "Lowering Your Cholesterol Levels" section in this chapter.

Table 10-1	Meaning of Claims on Food Labels
Claims for Cholesterol	**Description**
Free	Less than 2 mg per serving and 2 grams or less of saturated fat per serving.
Low	20 mg or less cholesterol and 2 grams or less saturated fat per serving.
Reduced or less	At least 25 percent less cholesterol and 2 grams or less saturated fat per serving than the original product.
Free	Less than 0.5 grams fat per serving.
Low	3 grams or less fat per serving.
Reduced or less	At least 25 percent less fat per serving than the original product.
Light	One-third fewer calories or 50 percent less fat per serving than the original product.
__% fat free	Meets the definition of "low fat" or "fat free" if stated as 100 percent fat free.
Claims for Saturated Fat	
Free	Less than 0.5 grams saturated fat per serving.
Low	1 gram or less saturated fat and no more than 15 percent of calories from saturated fat.
Reduced or less	At least 25 percent less saturated fat per serving than the original product.

(continued on following page)

Table 10-1 Meaning of Claims on Food Labels *(continued)*	
Claims for Cholesterol, Fat, and Saturated Fat	
Lean*	Less than 10 grams total fat, less than 4.5 grams saturated fat, and less than 95 mg cholesterol per 3-ounce serving and per 100 grams.
Extra Lean*	Less than 5 grams total fat, less than 2 grams saturated fat, and less than 95 mg cholesterol per 3-ounce serving and per 100 grams.

*On seafood, game meat, meat, and poultry.

The goal for the full day's diet should be to select foods that together add up to no more than 100 percent of the daily value for fat, saturated fat, and cholesterol. If you see a nutritional claim with the words "fat" or "cholesterol" on a package label, it is important to understand what that claim means. Ⓔ

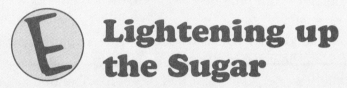

Chapter 11

Lightening up the Sugar

The average American consumes about 20.5 teaspoons, or nearly 3 ounces, of added sugar each day. That adds up to 68.5 pounds of added sugar or sugars that do not occur naturally in foods per year! As most of us know, there is absolutely nothing unusual about a craving for sweets. But in excess, these sugary foods can take a toll on our health.

What Is Sugar?

Sugar belongs to the carbohydrate group, which also includes starches and fibers. Starch and fiber are known as complex carbohydrates, and sugar is known as a simple carbohydrate. Carbohydrates are one of the three macronutrients that provide calories and energy in our diets, with the other two being fat and protein. Carbohydrates are our body's primary source of fuel or energy.

Both simple and complex carbohydrates provide 4 calories per gram, and both are broken down or metabolized into a blood sugar called "glucose." Our bodies use glucose for fuel or energy. The body cannot tell the difference between the different forms of sugar.

Traditional sweeteners, such as sugar and sugar alcohols, are referred to as "nutritive" sweeteners because they supply actual calories and therefore energy to the body. Artificial sweeteners, such as aspartame or saccharin, are referred to as "non-nutritive" sweeteners because they do not break down in the body and so do not supply calories and energy to the body.

Simple Sugars

Simple sugars are found naturally in milk and milk products in the form of lactose and in fruit in the form of fructose. Simple sugars are also found naturally in some vegetables in very small portions. These foods contain sugar but also contain loads of essential vitamins, minerals, and fiber.

Many simple carbohydrate foods contain refined sugars and few essential vitamins and minerals. Examples include molasses, maple syrup, table sugar, candy, soft drinks, cakes, and cookies. These foods are sometimes called "empty calorie" foods because they provide calories but very little or no nutritional value. Sugar can be part of a healthy diet if you are eating the correct balance of simple and complex carbohydrates and not loading up on the sweet stuff.

Simple carbohydrates or sugars are digested quickly because of their simple structure. In comparison, complex carbohydrates take longer to digest. This is because they have a more complex structure and are usually packed with fiber. Examples are vegetables, breads, cereals, legumes, and pasta.

All carbohydrates, whether simple or complex, are made of the same three elements: carbon, hydrogen, and oxygen. These three elements are arranged in single units to create different types of carbohydrates. For example, simple carbohydrates are made up of only one or two units, while starches (or complex carbohydrates) and fiber are made up of many more.

There are different types of simple sugars. Table sugar is only one type. Sugars with only one sugar unit are called "monosaccharides." Sugars with two sugar units are called "disaccharides." The three types of monosaccharides are fructose, galactose, and glucose.

When two of these are joined together they become disaccharides, as follows:

- Sucrose = glucose + fructose
- Lactose = glucose + galactose
- Maltose = glucose + glucose

Sucrose is another name for table sugar.

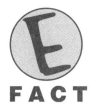

FACT

When checking the ingredient labels on packaged food, you will find all types of sweeteners listed. Any single ingredient that you find that ends in "-ose" is simply another word for a type of sugar.

In comparison, complex carbohydrates such as starches and fibers are called polysaccharides, meaning they are made up of many sugar units. They are longer chains of simple carbohydrates or sugar.

Sugar Alcohols

Sugar alcohols are used to sweeten foods. The "alcohol" in these sweeteners refers only to their structure; the foods themselves do not contain alcoholic beverages. Besides adding sweetness to foods, sugar alcohols also add texture to foods, help foods stay moist, and prevent browning when food is heated.

Sugar alcohols contain about 4 calories per gram, like sugar does, but they are absorbed more slowly and incompletely into the bloodstream.

Because sugar alcohols are not absorbed completely, they contribute slightly fewer calories to the body than sugar and do not promote tooth decay or cause a sudden spike in blood sugar. In comparison to regular sugar, they need little to no insulin for metabolism. They include sorbitol, xylitol, lactitol, mannitol, and maltitol and are used primarily to sweeten sugar-free candy, cookies, and chewing gums. The FDA classifies some of these sugar alcohols and others as "generally recognized as safe" (abbreviated as GRAS) as approved food additives.

How Much Sugar?

The typical American diet is packed with sugar, and most of it is hidden. Nutrition experts agree that Americans need to cut back. There is no current RDA for sugar, but experts recommend that about 55 to 60 percent of total calories in your diet should come from carbohydrates, with less than 10 percent coming from simple sugars. The bulk of carbohydrate choices should be complex carbohydrates, and most of the simple carbohydrate choices should come from fruits and dairy products, which also contain vitamins, minerals, and fiber.

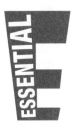

You should avoid making carbohydrate choices from refined foods high in sugar, the empty calorie foods, since they are usually low in the nutrients we need to maintain health and energy levels.

The USDA advises people who eat a 2,000-calorie healthful diet to try to limit themselves to about 10 teaspoons (40 grams) of added sugars per day. Many individual foods provide large fractions of the USDA's recommended sugar limits. For instance, a cup of regular ice cream provides 60 percent of a day's worth of added sugar, a 12-ounce Pepsi provides 103 percent, and a Hostess Lemon Fruit Pie provides 115 percent. Foods with refined sugars seem to frequently take the place of more nutritious alternatives, such as soft drinks instead of milk, juice, or water, or candy bars instead of fresh fruit. Experts often express concern that because less nutritious, sugary foods often replace more healthful foods, diets high in sugar can contribute to health problems such as osteoporosis, cancer, and heart disease.

Carbohydrates are broken down into glucose and used as energy. They are also stored in the muscles and liver as glycogen. When too many calories are consumed, with too many of them coming from sugar, sugar may be converted to body fat, which can lead to weight problems. Avoiding sugars alone will not correct an overweight problem. When trying to lose weight, reduce the total amount of calories from the food you eat and increase your level of physical activity.

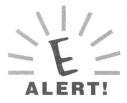

ALERT!

For some people, consuming large amounts of certain sugar alcohols can have a laxative effect. It is best to consume foods with these types of sweeteners in moderation in case you have a lower tolerance.

Too much sugar in the diet can promote tooth decay. A cavity is produced when bacteria, found in dental plaque in your mouth, mixes with carbohydrates, both sugar and starches, and makes acids. These acids can eat away at your tooth enamel, causing tooth decay or dental caries. Frequent between-meal snacking on foods high in sugar and starches seems to have the biggest impact on the formation of dental caries. Sucking on hard candy or slowly sipping a soft drink all day covers your teeth with plaque all day. Since the whole process continues for about twenty to thirty minutes, it is important to floss and brush your teeth with fluoride toothpaste as soon as you can after eating carbohydrates. This can help remove the plaque and food particles. The longer these foods are in your mouth, the higher your risk for dental caries and/or tooth decay.

Curbing Your Sugar Intake

If consumed in moderation, sugar can be part of a healthy diet. People who want to reduce their added sugar intake should eat more nutrient-rich whole grains, vegetables, fruits, and sources of lean protein. Changing a habit takes time, so give yourself at least two weeks to get used to eating less sugar and to calm your sweet tooth.

Follow some of these helpful hints to help cut down on your sugar intake:

- Watch your portion sizes when eating sugary foods. Share a dessert with a friend, or eat a miniature instead of a regular-size candy bar.
- When you feel that sweet tooth coming on, get in the habit of reaching for healthier foods. Try foods such as fruit, flavored yogurt, or fruit juice.
- Get in the habit of reading labels. Products you thought might contain little sugar may actually be loaded with it. Fat-free foods are a good example. They may be fat-free, but they are *not* calorie-free and may get most of the calories from added sugar.
- Break the soft-drink habit. Regular soft drinks are loaded with sugar. Better choices are water, low-fat or fat-free milk, or fruit juice. Be sure fruit juices are 100 percent pure fruit juice.
- If you drink more than 2 cups of coffee or 2 cans of soda each day, try to cut back. Caffeine can increase your craving for sugar.
- Gradually cut back on the sugar in your recipes. The rule of thumb for cakes and cakelike cookies is to reduce the sugar to half a cup for every cup of flour called for in the recipe. For muffins and quick breads, you need at least 1 tablespoon sugar for every cup of flour. For yeast breads, use only 1 teaspoon of sugar for every cup of flour used.
- Try using sugar substitutes in your coffee, tea, or on your cereal. They add flavor and very few calories. Be careful to moderate your use of sugar substitutes, though, because you will not actually be teaching yourself to curb your tastes for sweets.
- Allow yourself one planned sweet treat everyday. You won't deny your desire for sweets, but you can keep the cravings under control by planning for them in advance.
- Keep a diary. Note the times you crave sweets, where you are, what you are doing, how you are feeling, and how you deal with it. Use the diary to learn what steps you need to take to curb your sweet tooth.

People commonly eat processed foods without realizing how much sugar is in the food. Just about every food contains some sugar, but some sugars are added and some are natural. The biggest source of added sugars is nondiet soft drinks, accounting for one-third of added sugars consumed. Other large sources are sugar-coated breakfast cereals and sweet desserts. As manufacturers add more sugars to more products, people are becoming more expectant of and more adapted to a sweeter taste.

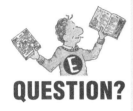

QUESTION?

Can you be addicted to sugar?
No. The term "sugar addiction" describes a sweet tooth. An actual addiction is defined as either an emotional and/or physical dependence that includes symptoms of withdrawal. This does not happen with sugar. A sweet tooth or craving for sweets is actually a learned behavior from eating lots of sweets over time. It can be unlearned by changing your behavior.

If a food has one of the following terms listed first or second in its list of ingredients, it is likely to be higher in sugar: brown sugar, corn sweetener, corn syrup, fructose, fruit juice concentrate, glucose (dextrose), high-fructose corn syrup, honey, invert sugar, lactose, maltose, molasses, raw sugar, table sugar (sucrose), or syrup.

Sugar Myths

Eating too much sugar is not the cause for hyperactivity or deficit disorder in children. There is no scientifically proven link between sugar intake and these types of disorders.

Nor does eating too much sugar cause diabetes. Diabetes is a disorder in which the body cannot properly regulate sugar levels. The causes of diabetes are not yet fully understood, but factors that definitely play a role include genetics, obesity, illness, and age. Although food is used in managing diabetes, along with physical activity and sometimes medications, food is not what causes diabetes.

Sugar does not cause hypoglycemia or low blood sugar. Hypoglycemia is a condition that causes blood sugar levels to drop below normal between meals. Hypoglycemia, which occurs about two to four hours after eating, is the result of too much insulin being released. The excess insulin causes a drop in blood sugar, which in turn may result in shaking, rapid heartbeat, and perspiration. It's important to differentiate hypoglycemia from hunger, which can also cause some of these symptoms. Many people tend to self-diagnose, thinking they have hypoglycemia, but it is actually a fairly rare condition. The best advice is to track your symptoms along with the times you eat. Give this information to your doctor so he or she can diagnose you properly.

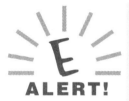

We tend to think that fat-free or lower-fat foods are healthy because all or some of the fat has been taken out. The problem is that manufacturers usually take the fat out and then make up for the taste by adding extra sugar. If you think you don't eat much sugar, make sure you are taking a look at those labels.

Eating too much sugar is not the single cause of weight gain. Eating too many calories from all foods, including carbohydrates, fats, and proteins, is what can causes you to gain extra pounds.

Nutrition and health experts have concluded that tooth decay is the only health problem with a direct relationship to sugar. In moderation, sugar can be a part of a healthy diet, making nutritious foods more appealing by adding taste, texture, aroma, and color.

Artificial Sweeteners

There is a long history of controversy concerning sugar substitutes, or non-nutritive sweeteners. These types of sweeteners, also known as "intense sweeteners," sweeten with little volume. The United States leads the world in consumption of high-intensity sweeteners, with responsibility for approximately 50 percent of the world demand. These sweeteners can be very effective sugar substitutes for people with diabetes who cannot tolerate regular sugar. Sugar substitutes can also be helpful to people on a weight reduction program.

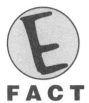

FACT

The American Dietetic Association holds that consumers can safely enjoy a wide range of nutritive and non-nutritive sweeteners when they are consumed in moderation and within the context of a diet consistent with the Dietary Guidelines for Americans.

Four artificial sweeteners have been approved for use in the United States: aspartame, saccharin, acesulfame-K, and sucralose.

Aspartame

Aspartame is 160 to 220 times sweeter than table sugar. It was first discovered in 1965, when it was marketed as NutraSweet and Equal. This intense sweetener is made up of two amino acids: phenylalanine and aspartic acid. Since first approving aspartame in 1981, the FDA has evaluated aspartame twenty-six times. In 1996, the FDA approved aspartame as a general-purpose sweetener for use in all foods and beverages. Aspartame is also approved for use in more than 100 other countries. Because aspartame contains phenylalanine, people with phenylketonuria (PKU) need to be cautious about consuming too many foods and beverages sweetened with aspartame.

Aspartame in included in some common foods in the following amounts:

- Up to 225 mg in a 12-ounce diet soft drink
- 100 mg in an 8-ounce drink made from powder
- 80 mg in an 8-ounce yogurt
- Up to 32 mg in ¾ cup sweetened cereal
- Up to 47 mg in ½ cup frozen dairy dessert

Packets of aspartame, for sweetening foods at the table, contain 37 mg aspartame, equivalent to 2 teaspoons of sugar. In the granular form. 1 teaspoon of aspartame weighs 16 mg, with the sweetening power of 1 teaspoon of sugar.

Aspartame can lose its sweetness when heated for a long period of time. Therefore, when you use aspartame in cooking, add it after the foods are cooked.

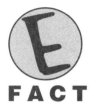

FACT

Phenylketonuria, or PKU, is a rare genetic disorder that keeps the body from properly metabolizing the amino acid phenylalanine. This can cause toxic effects in the body. All babies are tested for this disorder at birth. If you have this disorder, you should consult your doctor before using aspartame.

Saccharin

Saccharin was discovered over 100 years ago and is 300 times sweeter than table sugar. Today it is used in soft drinks and tabletop sweeteners, such as Sweet'N Low. The FDA proposed a ban on saccharin in 1977 because a few studies showed that when taken in very large amounts, it seemed to cause cancer in laboratory rats. In 1991 the FDA lifted the ban and now considers saccharin to be safe as a food additive on an interim basis for use in cosmetics, foods and beverages, pharmaceuticals, tabletop sugar substitutes, and in chewing gum.

It would be extremely difficult to consume the amounts given to the laboratory rats from foods alone. The amount of saccharin must appear on the food label and is limited to no more than 12 mg per ounce in beverages—20 mg per sweetening equivalent in 1 teaspoon of sugar—or no more than 30 mg per serving of food. The warning still remains on product labels. Unlike aspartame, saccharin does not lose its sweetness when heated, so it can be used in cooked and baked goods. However, because it does not have the same bulk as sugar, it may not work well in all types of recipes.

Acesulfame-K

Acesulfame-K is 200 times sweeter than table sugar. The "K" in the name stands for the mineral potassium. It can be found in candies, baked goods, desserts, soft drinks, and tabletop sweeteners such as Sweet One. Acesulfame-K is a newer artificial sweetener. It was approved by the FDA for use in the United States in 1988 and is marketed under the brand name "Sunette." Acesulfame-K is heat stable, so it can be used in cooking and baking. But because it does not have the same bulk as sugar, it may not work well in all recipes.

Sucralose

Sucralose is 600 times sweeter than sugar. Sucralose provides no energy; it is not well absorbed and is excreted in the urine essentially unchanged. Sucralose is one of the most recently approved artificial sweeteners. It was approved in April 1998 as a tabletop sweetener and for use in a number of desserts, confections, and nonalcoholic beverages. The FDA concluded from a review of more than 110 studies in humans and animals that sucralose does not pose a carcinogenic, reproductive, or neurological risk to humans. This sweetener is heat stable and therefore can be used in cooking and baking.

More sweeteners are in line to be approved by the FDA and introduced on the market soon.

Are Artificial Sweeteners Safe?

Artificial sweeteners that are approved by the FDA are considered safe for use in moderation. They can be part of a healthy lifestyle. The FDA puts sweeteners through extensive testing before considering them safe for the general population.

Some sweeteners are considered "generally recognized as safe" (or GRAS) ingredients, and others are considered food additives. The 1958 Food Additives Amendment to the Food, Drug, and Cosmetic Act defined these terms. GRAS substances are those whose use is generally recognized by experts as safe, based on their extensive history of use in food before 1958 or on published scientific evidence.

Examples of substances that are classified as GRAS include salt, sugar, spices, vitamins, and monosodium glutamate (MSG). If at any time new evidence or research suggests that a GRAS substance may be unsafe for human consumption, federal authorities have the power to prohibit its use or require further studies of its safety. The 1958 amendment also states that the FDA must approve the safety of all additives.

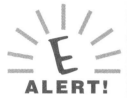

ALERT!

The American Dietetic Association states that "intense sweeteners within FDA guidelines are safe by use of pregnant women. But if you are pregnant or breastfeeding you may want to check with your doctor before consuming any products with artificial sweeteners."

The safety of food additives is expressed as Acceptable Daily Intake (ADI), or the estimated amount per kilogram of body weight that a person can safely consume every day over a lifetime without health risk. The ADI is a conservative level: it reflects an amount 100 times less than the maximum level at which no adverse health risks are observed in animal studies (and, very occasionally, human studies). The ADI is used by the FDA and the Joint Expert Committee of Food Additions (JECFA) of the United Nations Food and Agricultural Organization and the World Health Organization.

Table 11-1	Acceptable Daily Intake for FDA-Approved Non-Nutritive Sweeteners
Sweetener	**ADI**
Aspartame	50 mg/ kilogram body weight*
Saccharin	5 mg/ kilogram body weight*
AcesulfameK	15 mg/ kilogram body weight*
Sucralose	0 to 15mg/ kilogram body weight*

*Weight in pounds divided by 2.2 will equal kilograms of body weight.

Foods that contain artificial or intense sweeteners are not really intended for infants or young children. These sweeteners are safe for children, but at such a young age they need calories to sustain their rapid growth spurts. Parents should limit their young children's intake of saccharin; data is inadequate concerning its use in children.

Sugar and Diabetes

The American Diabetic Association estimates that 16 million Americans suffer from diabetes. Diabetes is a disease in which the body does not produce or properly use insulin. Insulin is a hormone made in the pancreas that is needed to convert sugar, starches, and other food into energy needed for daily life. People with diabetes have trouble controlling their blood sugar levels because their body does not properly produce or use insulin. As a result, blood sugar, or glucose, accumulates in the blood and makes blood sugar levels rise. Instead of being used for energy as it should be, sugar passes out of the body through the urine. This puts an extra strain on the kidneys, causing frequent urination and excessive thirst. The cause of diabetes is a mystery, although genetic and environmental factors such as obesity and lack of exercise seem to play definite roles.

Types of Diabetes

There are three types of diabetes. In **Type 1** diabetes, the pancreas produces no insulin. This type can occur in anyone but occurs most often in children and young adults, accounting for only about 5 to 10 percent of diabetes. Its main cause is genetic. Type 1 diabetics must take daily insulin injections for survival.

Type 2 diabetes is a metabolic disorder in which the body does not properly make or use insulin. It is the most common form of diabetes, accounting for 90 to 95 percent of the disease. Being overweight or obese is a common risk factor for this type of diabetes. It can usually be controlled through diet and exercise though it is nearing epidemic proportions. This is due to an increased number of older Americans and a greater prevalence of obesity and sedentary lifestyles.

Type 3 diabetes is gestational diabetes, which can occur during pregnancy. It is usually the result of changing hormones within the woman's body. It needs to be carefully controlled throughout the pregnancy and usually disappears once the baby is born. Women who have gestational diabetes are at a higher risk of developing it in later pregnancies.

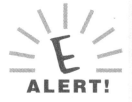

ALERT!

Uncontrolled diabetes can cause major health problems and can even be life threatening. It is a major risk factor for heart disease, poor circulation, eye disorders, foot problems, and kidney disorders. In addition to taking your diabetes medication or insulin as instructed by your doctor, you can have a positive influence on your blood sugar and your health by choosing foods wisely, being physically active, and reducing your stress levels.

Sugar Guidelines

The American Diabetes Association has changed its guidelines to be more flexible so that they meet more individual needs. They now say diabetics may eat sugar in an occasional piece of pie or a cookie or two, as long as they closely monitor their blood sugar for unhealthy surges. According to the new 2002 nutrition guidelines, the kind of carbohydrates diabetics eat is not as important as how much they're eating. When it comes to affecting blood sugar, a carbohydrate is a carbohydrate, whether starch or sugar, and the body treats all of them the same way. Researchers have found that sugar does not raise blood sugar levels any more rapidly than starches do. However, this does not mean that all diabetics can go ahead and eat all sweets. Some are heavy in saturated fats and loaded with calories and are not practical for an overweight diabetic. Eating more complex carbohydrates and natural sugars adds more nutrition to the diet. Most diabetics don't have to make radical changes in their diets as long as they eat a healthy and balanced diet, test blood sugars regularly, are physically active, and take their insulin or medication as directed.

Glycemic Index

The glycemic index is a rating system that predicts how quickly a specific food will affect the blood sugar. Not all carbohydrates are equal in how quickly they raise blood glucose. The glycemic index uses a scale of numbers for foods with carbohydrates that have the slowest to highest effects on blood sugar. Two indexes are in use. One uses a scale of 1 to 100, with 100 representing a glucose tablet, which has the most rapid effect on blood sugar. The other common index uses a scale with 100 representing white bread; in this scale, some foods will be above 100.

The glycemic index reflects the rankings of single foods. Factors that influence a food's glycemic index include the food's type of fiber, the presence of fat, the form of sugar in the food, and the effects of protein and fat eaten with the food. All of these factors will slow the absorption rate of sugar into the blood.

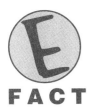

FACT

The numbers attributed to each carbohydrate-rich food are not additive. In other words, adding All Bran cereal (with an index of 49) to a banana (index of 61) does not equal 110.

The glycemic index is not recommended for use as a complete dietary guide because it does not provide nutritional guidelines for all foods. It is simply an indication of how the metabolism will respond to carbohydrates. Some experts believe it is too complicated to be practical and that simply tracking carbohydrates, eating healthily, and maintaining a healthy weight is sufficient. Consult a registered dietitian if you are a diabetic and are interested in using the glycemic index.

Sugar Label Lingo

To eat sugars in moderation, it is important to understand and know their sources. The food label or nutrition claims on packaged foods can clue you in to how much sugar is in the product. The food label lists total carbohydrates and sugar in grams per serving. Sugar is part of the total carbohydrate amount listed. Check for foods that provide plenty of nutrients such as fiber, vitamins, and minerals, along with sugar. If you see a nutritional claim that includes the word "sugar," it is important to understand what that claims means. The following describes some of those claims:

- **Calorie free:** less than 5 calories
- **Sugar free:** less than 0.5 grams sugar per serving
- **Reduced sugar or less sugar:** at least 25 percent less sugar or sugars per serving, as compared with a standard serving size
- **No added sugars, without added sugars, no sugar:** no sugars added during processing or packing, including ingredients that contain sugar, such as juice or dry fruit
- **Low sugar:** may not be used as a claim on food labels

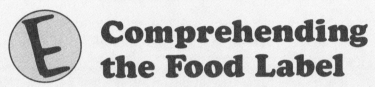

Chapter 12

Comprehending the Food Label

L earning how to properly read food labels enables you to make smarter nutrition choices on the foods that you buy. The food label provides you with relevant information on essential nutrients and ingredients. It is well worth your time to learn how to interpret food labels and how to put them to work for you and your health!

What Is on the Food Label?

The two leading U.S. food label authorities are the Food Safety and Inspection Services (FSIS), which is part of the U.S. Department of Agriculture, and the Food and Drug Administration (FDA), which is part of the U.S. Department of Health and Human Services. The FSIS regulates labeling on meat and poultry products, while the FDA regulates the labeling and ingredients of just about all other food products.

Food labels are required on most prepared foods such as bread, cereal, canned and frozen foods, snacks, desserts, and drinks. Nutrition labeling is voluntary on fruits, vegetables, meat, poultry, and fish. Nutrition labels are not required on foods that contain few significant nutrients, such as coffee and tea, or on certain ready-to-eat foods such as unpackaged deli foods, bakery items, and restaurant foods.

Food labels contain up to four different types of useful nutritional information to help you make healthier choices:

1. The Nutrition Facts Panel is the square box on the food label that provides detailed information on calories and essential nutrients such as fat, sodium, cholesterol, fiber, and several vitamins and minerals. The Nutrition Facts Panel is required to appear on almost all food labels.
2. The ingredient list that appears on packaged foods provides a detailed overview of product ingredients. The ingredient list must appear on all foods labels of foods with more than one ingredient.
3. Nutrition claims or nutrition descriptions can help you to quickly and easily find foods that meet your specific nutritional goals. These include claims such as "low fat," "cholesterol free," "high fiber," and "low sodium." Nutrition claims are not required on labels.
4. Health claims describe the potential health benefits of a specific food or nutrient within the food. These include claims such as that for calcium, which states its benefit for reducing osteoporosis, or folic acid, which reduces the risk of neural tube birth defects. Health claims are not required on labels.

The Nutrition Facts Panel

The Nutrition Facts Panel provides key nutritional information. At its top is the serving size, servings per container, calories per serving, and calories from fat. Below that is a list of the three macronutrients as well as other important nutrients. These nutrients are listed in grams or milligrams.

Below those are listed a few micronutrients, two vitamins, and two minerals, which are displayed in percentages. On the right side of the label is a column headed "Percent Daily Value." Near the bottom of the label is a footnote stating that the Percent Daily Values are based on a 2,000-calorie diet that includes a list of Daily Reference Values.

FIGURE 12-1
Nutrition
Food Label

Servings per container refer to the number of servings found in this container.

Amount per serving refers to the nutrient content for each serving of food.

This section lists the recommended daily limits of fat, saturated fat, cholesterol, and sodium, plus amounts of carbohydrates and fiber one should aim for on a daily basis for diets of 2,000 and 2,500 calories.

Nutrition Facts

Serving Size 1/2 cup (114 g)
Servings Per Container 4

Amount Per Serving

Calories: 90   Calories from Fat 30

	% Daily Value*
Total Fat 3g	5%
Saturated Fat 0g	0%
Cholesterol 0mg	0%
Sodium 300mg	13%
Total Carbohydrate 13g	4%
Dietary Fiber 3g	12%
Sugars 3g	
Protein 3g	

Vitamin A 80%	Vitamin C 60%
Calcium 4% •	Iron 4%

* Percent Daily Values are based on a 2,000-calorie diet. Your daily values may be higher or lower depending on your calorie needs:

	Calories: 2,000	2,500
Total Fat	Less than 65g	80g
Saturated Fat	Less than 20g	25g
Cholesterol	Less than 300mg	300mg
Sodium	Less than 2,400mg	2,400mg
Total Carbohydrate	300mg	375mg
Dietary Fiber	25g	30g

Calories per gram
Fat 9 • Carbohydrate 4 • Protein 4

The **serving size** refers to the average amount or portion a person should eat at one time.

% Daily Value is based on a 2,000-calorie daily diet. These values may be higher or lower based on the number of calories in one's diet. One should aim for 100% each day of total carbohydrate, dietary fiber, vitamins, and minerals and not exceed 100% for total fat, sodium and cholesterol.

Serving Size

The place to start when looking at the Nutrition Facts Panel is the serving size and the number of servings in the package. Serving sizes are provided in familiar units, such as cups, tablespoons, or pieces, followed by the metric measure. The serving sizes are based on the amounts of food that people normally eat, making it more realistic and easier to compare with similar foods. The serving size is the first item you should look at; *all* the nutrition information on the label pertains to the serving size stated on the label.

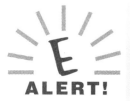

Be aware that if you purchase a product because you feel it is low in a nutrient such as fat or calories, you should make sure the serving size is something you will realistically eat. If you don't follow the serving size, it may not be low in that nutrient anymore.

On the sample label shown in **FIGURE 12-1**, the serving size is ½ cup, and there are four servings per container. That means that all the information pertains to ½ cup. If you ate the whole container, you would need to multiply all of the information on the label by four.

Calories and Calories from Fat

Calories per serving measures how much energy you would receive from a single serving of a food. The label also provides the number of calories in one serving that come from fat. In the example label, there are 90 calories in a serving, and there are 30 calories from fat. This means that out of the total 90 calories per serving, 30 (or a third of them) are coming from fat. We know that calories in food only come from three sources: fat, protein, and carbohydrate. So this also tells you that the other 60 calories are coming from protein and/or carbohydrate sources. Now, if you ate the whole package, you would consume a total of four servings of the food, or 360 calories, with 120 calories from fat.

Nutrients on the Label

The specific nutrients listed on the Nutrition Facts Panel were selected because of their relationship to current health issues. Nutrients that are required on all food labels include total fat, saturated fat, cholesterol, sodium, total carbohydrate, dietary fiber, sugar, protein, vitamin A, vitamin C, calcium, and iron. Manufacturers can add additional nutrients, but the ones listed are required. Americans generally consume too much of the first four nutrients on the list.

The total fat content consists of both types of fat: saturated and unsaturated (polyunsaturated and monounsaturated). Under total fat, these fats are separated out. Only saturated fat is required to be listed; unsaturated can be listed but is not required. Saturated fat is required because people should be aware of their intake. Lowering your intake of saturated fat can decrease your risk of heart disease.

Cholesterol and sodium are the other two nutrients that most Americans generally consume too much of. Lowering cholesterol can benefit heart health, and for some people, lowering sodium can help decrease the risk for high blood pressure. Both of these nutrients are measured in milligrams.

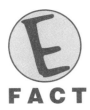

FACT

Most Americans do not get enough dietary fiber, vitamin A, vitamin C, calcium, or iron. Including enough of these nutrients in your daily diet can help improve health and reduce the risk of some diseases and conditions.

The two vitamins and minerals on the list are referenced as Reference Daily Intakes (RDIs). The RDI values are established by the Food and Drug Administration (FDA) and are used only on food labels. Initially the values on food labels were based on the highest 1968 RDA for each nutrient, to ensure that needs for all groups were met. RDI replaces the term "U.S. RDA," which was introduced in 1973 as a label reference value for vitamins, minerals, and protein in voluntary nutrition labeling. The name change was completed because of confusion that existed over U.S. RDAs—the FDA values used on food labels—and RDAs. The RDIs were put into effect when the new food labels emerged in 1992.

The food label should be used to help limit those nutrients you should cut back on and to increase those nutrients you should consume more of.

Percent Daily Value

The nutrients on food labels are expressed in two distinct ways: in terms of the amount by weight per serving, using grams or milligrams, or in terms of Percent Daily Value. The Percent Daily Value is an estimate of how a serving of the food meets the daily requirement for each nutrient, based on a 2,000-calorie diet. This is meant to help you decide whether a specific nutrient in a serving of food contributes a lot or a little to your total daily intake. Your daily goal should be to meet 100 percent or less of the daily value for nutrients; you should be consuming less fat, saturated fat, sodium, sugar, and cholesterol. Likewise, your goal should be to get at least 100 percent or more of nutrients you should be consuming more of, such as fiber, complex carbohydrates, calcium, iron, vitamin A, and vitamin C.

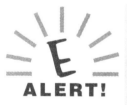

ALERT!

Be careful not to be confused by Percent Daily Values. The value does *not* indicate how much a nutrient is in a food. It simply means how the food, per serving, compares to your total daily nutritional intake. For example, if a food states 5 percent daily value for fat, that does *not* mean there is 5 percent fat in the product. It *does* mean that the product is using up 5 percent of your daily fat needs for the day.

Personalized Calorie Levels

If you consume less or more than 2,000 calories, the daily value can be adjusted for your specific calorie level. Use **TABLE 12-1** to find out how you can adjust the total Percent Daily Values for specific calorie levels. If you were on a 1,600-calorie diet—20 percent less than the standard 2,000 calories—you would figure your daily value to total only 80 percent for the day, a 20-percent reduction. The nutrients you would adjust are total fat, saturated fat, carbohydrate, and dietary fiber. Cholesterol and sodium are always the same amount, no matter how many calories you ingest, so figure for these to always add up to 100 percent each day.

To find out your recommended amounts for certain nutrients for your personalized calorie intake, follow the values in **TABLE 12-2**.

Even though you may not know exactly how many calories you eat in a day, you can still use the Percent Daily Value as a frame of reference.

Table 12-1   Adjusted Percent Daily Value for Specific Calorie Levels

Calories	Adjusted Percent Daily Value
1,400	70 percent
1,600	80 percent
2,000	100 percent
2,200	110 percent
2,500	125 percent
2,800	140 percent
3,200	160 percent

Table 12-2   Recommended Amounts of Nutrients Based on Calorie Intake

Nutrient	Calories*						
	1,400	1,600	2,000	2,200	2,500	2,800	3,200
Total Fat (g)	47	53	65	73	80	93	107
Saturated Fat (g)	16	18	20	24	25	31	36
Cholesterol (mg)	300	300	300	300	300	300	300
Sodium (mg)	2,400	2,400	2,400	2,400	2,400	2,400	2,400
Total carbohydrate (g)	210	240	300	330	375	420	480
Dietary fiber** (g)	20	20	25	25	30	32	37

*These calorie levels may not apply to children and adolescents, who have changing calorie requirements. For specific advice concerning personal calorie levels, consult your doctor or a registered dietitian.

**20 grams is the minimum amount of fiber recommended for all calorie levels below 2,000.

How Percent Daily Value Is Calculated

The Percent Daily Values are calculated using the reference values in the footnote of each food label. These values are the same on every food label. The daily reference values listed are calculated based on both a 2,000- and a 2,500-calorie diet. The daily values that are actually listed on the label use the Daily Reference Intake values for the 2,000-calorie diet.

Do you need to know how to calculate percentages to follow this advice? No, the Percent Daily Value does the math for you. It helps you to interpret what the amounts mean (grams and milligrams) by placing them all on the same type of scale (0–100 Percent Daily Value). This helps you tell high from low and understand which nutrients may be contributing a lot or a little to your daily recommended allowance.

The daily value amount of the nutrient, per serving, is calculated by dividing the reference value to see how much of your nutrient allotment is used up for the day. The following example illustrates how to calculate daily value for a food containing 3 grams of fat per serving:

1. The sample label lists 3 grams of fat per serving.
2. The reference value for fat, found in the footnote of the label, is 65 grams per day (based on a 2,000-calorie diet).
3. Divide 3 grams by 65 grams to equal 0.046 or 4.6 percent. Rounded up, this is 5 percent. If you look at the sample label, 5 percent is the Percent Daily Value for fat.
4. This means that when you eat a serving of this product, it is using up 5 percent of the fat you are allowed for a day, based on a 2,000-calorie diet, or 5 percent of the 65 grams of fat. In other words, you have 95 percent of your fat allowance left for the day.

Expressing nutrients as a percentage of the Daily Values is intended to help prevent misinterpretations that can arise with quantitative values. For example, a food that contains 150 mg of sodium could seem high in sodium just because the number 150 seems relatively large. In actuality, however, 150 mg is only about 6 percent of the daily value for sodium, which is 2,400 mg per day. On the other hand, a food with 5 grams of saturated fat could be construed as being low in that nutrient; however, that food would provide 25 percent of the total daily value for saturated fat (20 g).

Sugar and Protein

Sugars and protein do not have a Percent Daily Value on the Nutrition Facts Panel. Sugar has no daily reference value because no recommendations have been made for the total amount of sugars to eat in a day. The sugar on the label includes naturally occurring sugars, such as those in fruit and dairy products, as well as added sugars, such as those in soft drinks and baked goods. Check the ingredient list to find more information on added sugars.

You will not always see a Percent Daily Value for protein. It is only required if a claim is made for protein, such as "high in protein," or if the food is specifically meant for use by infants and children under four years old. The government has decided that current scientific evidence indicates that protein intake is not a public health concern for adults or for children over four years. Protein needs are more individualized and should really be based on an individual's weight and physical activity.

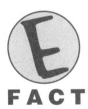

FACT

If the Percent Daily Value of protein is required, it is calculated as 10 percent of total calorie intake. On a 2,000-calorie diet, this would equal 50 grams of protein. The minimum amount of protein recommended for all calorie levels is 46 grams.

Quick Guide to Percent Daily Values

To help you quickly decide whether a food is high or low in a nutrient, use this general guide:

- **Low:** The food contains 5 percent or less of the daily value for a particular nutrient in a serving.
- **Good source:** One serving of a food contains 10 to 19 percent of the daily value for a particular nutrient.

- **High:** The food contains 20 percent or more of the daily value for a particular nutrient in a serving.
- **More:** A serving of food, altered or not, contains a nutrient that is at least 10 percent of the daily value more than the reference food. The 10 percent of daily value also applies to claims of "fortified," "enriched," "added," "extra," and "plus"; but in those cases, the food must be altered.

This means that 5 percent or less of a daily value would be considered low for all nutrients that you want to limit, such as fat, saturated fat, cholesterol, and sodium. This also means that 20 percent or more of the daily value would be considered high for those nutrients that you want to consume in greater amounts, such as fiber, calcium, iron, vitamin A, and vitamin C.

Footnote to the Food Label

The asterisk used after the heading "Percent Daily Value" refers to the footnote in the lower part of the nutrition label. This section tells you that Percent Daily Values are based on recommendations for a 2,000-calorie diet and that your daily values may be higher or lower, depending on your calorie needs. This statement is required on all food labels. The remaining information in the full footnote, including the daily reference values for 2,000- and 2,500-calorie diets, as well as the calories per gram of the three macronutrients, may not be on the package if the label is small. When the full footnote does appear on a label, it will always be exactly the same. It doesn't change from product to product because it shows dietary advice for all Americans, not information about a specific food product.

Nutritional Claims

Labels often contain claims of desirable levels of individual nutrients. Regulations now strictly spell out what terms may be used to describe the level of a nutrient in a food and how those terms can be used. Nutrition claims can be used as another valuable tool that can help you to choose foods that are lower in calories, fat, cholesterol, and sodium and higher in fiber, vitamins, and minerals.

Some of the general claims used include the following:

- **Free:** A product contains none or only trivial amounts of one or more of these components: fat, saturated fat, cholesterol, sodium, sugars, and calories. For example, "calorie-free" means fewer than 5 calories per serving, and "sugar-free" and "fat-free" both mean less than 0.5 gram per serving. Other names for "free" that can be used include "without," "no," and "zero." (Skim milk can also be labeled "fat-free.")
- **Low:** Indicates foods that can be eaten frequently without exceeding dietary guidelines for one or more of these components: fat, saturated fat, cholesterol, sodium, and calories. Other terms that can be used include "low in," "contains small amount," "few," "low source," and "little."
- **Reduced:** A product that has been nutritionally altered contains at least 25 percent less of a nutrient or of calories than the regular, or reference, product. A reduced claim cannot be placed on a product if its reference food already meets the requirement for a "low" nutritional claim. Other words for reduced include "reduced in," "less," "lower," "lower in," and "fewer."

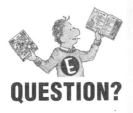

QUESTION?

How can a food label state "no added sugar" and then list sugar in grams on the Nutrition Facts Panel?
The sugar category on the panel includes both added and naturally occurring sugars. Some naturally occurring sugars are present in foods like fruit and milk products. So some products may contain naturally occurring sugar but not contain added sugar.

- **Less**: A food, altered or not, that contains 25 percent less of a nutrient or calories than its reference food. For example, pretzels that have 25 percent less fat than potato chips could carry a "less" claim. "Fewer" is an acceptable synonym.
- **Lean or extra lean**: Describes the fat content of meat, poultry,

seafood, and game meats. Lean means less than 10 grams fat, 4.5 grams or less saturated fat, and less than 95 mg cholesterol per serving and per 100 grams. Extra lean means less than 5 grams fat, less than 2 grams saturated fat, and less than 95 mg cholesterol per serving and per 100 grams.

- **Percent fat free**: A product bearing this claim must be a low-fat or a fat-free product. In addition, the claim must accurately reflect the amount of fat present in 100 grams of the food. Thus, if a food contains 2.5 grams fat per 50 grams, the claim must be "95 percent fat free."

- **Light**: This descriptor can mean two things. First, that a nutritionally altered product contains one-third fewer calories or half the fat of the reference food. If the food derives 50 percent or more of its calories from fat, the reduction must be 50 percent of the fat. Second, it can mean that the sodium content of a low-calorie, low-fat food has been reduced by 50 percent. In addition, the claim "light in sodium" may be used when the sodium content has been reduced by at least 50 percent.

Health Claims

Health claims on packaged foods are all approved and must be scientifically validated by the FDA. These types of claims describe a relationship between a specific nutrient or food substance and a disease or health-related condition. All of these claims must state the words "may" or "might" help prevent. Eleven claims are now approved for use on food labels:

1. **Calcium and osteoporosis:** Food must contain 20 percent or more of the daily value for calcium (200 mg) per serving, have a calcium content that equals or exceeds the food's phosphorus content, and contain a form of calcium that can be readily absorbed and used by the body.

2. **Fat and cancer:** Food must meet the nutrient content claim requirements for "low-fat" and for fish and game meats requirements for "extra-lean."

3. **Saturated fat and cholesterol and coronary heart disease (CHD):**
   Food must meet the definitions for the nutrient content claim "low
   saturated fat," "low-cholesterol," and "low-fat," or, for fish and game
   meats, for "extra-lean." It may mention the link between reduced risk
   of CHD and lower-saturated fat and cholesterol intakes to lower blood
   cholesterol levels.

4. **Fiber-containing grain products, fruits and vegetables, and cancer:**
   Food must be or must contain a grain product, fruit, or vegetable and
   meet the nutrient content claim requirements for "low-fat," and,
   without fortification, be a "good source" of dietary fiber.

5. **Fruits, vegetables, and grain products that contain fiber and risk
   of CHD:** Food must be or must contain fruits, vegetables, and grain
   products. It also must meet the nutrient content claim requirements
   for "low-saturated fat," "low-cholesterol," and "low-fat" and contain,
   without fortification, at least 0.6 grams soluble fiber per serving.

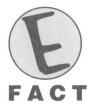

FACT

Many companies use health claims as marketing tools, but their
purpose is actually to help consumers make informed decisions
based on accepted scientific claims.

6. **Sodium and high blood pressure:** To carry this particular claim, a
   food must meet the nutrient content claim requirements for a "low-
   sodium" food.

7. **Fruits and vegetables and cancer:** Fruits and/or vegetables must meet
   the nutrient content claim requirements for "low-fat" and that, without
   fortification, for "good source" of at least one of the following: dietary
   fiber, vitamin A, or vitamin C. This claim relates diets low in fat and
   rich in fruits and vegetables to the reduced risk for cancer.

8. **Folic acid and neural tube defects:** This claim can be used on
   dietary supplements that contain sufficient amounts of folate and on
   conventional foods that are naturally good sources of folate, as long
   as they do not provide more than 100 percent of the daily value for
   vitamin A, preformed vitamin A, or vitamin D. An example of this
   claim is "Healthful diets with adequate folate may reduce a woman's

risk of having a child with a brain or spinal cord defect."

9. **Dietary sugar alcohols and dental caries (cavities):** This claim basically applies to products, such as candy or gum, that contain the sugar alcohols xylitol, sorbitol, mannitol, maltitol, isomalt, lactitol, hydrogenated starch hydrolysates, hydrogenated glucose syrups, or any combination of these. Besides the food's ingredients relationship to dental caries, the claim must also state that that "frequent between-meal consumption of foods high in sugars and starches promotes tooth decay."

10. **Soluble fiber from certain foods, such as whole oats and psyllium seed husk, and heart disease:** Package must also state that fiber needs to be part of a diet low in saturated fat and cholesterol and that the food must provide sufficient amounts of soluble fiber. The amount of soluble fiber in a serving of the food must be listed on the Nutrition Facts Panel.

11. **Soy protein and risk of coronary heart disease:** Food must have at least 6.25 grams of soy protein per reference amount and be low in saturated fat, cholesterol, and total fat.

Ingredient Lists

Food label information is not limited to health claims, nutritional claims, nutritional content, or daily value. Ingredients must also be listed on packaged foods that contain more than one ingredient. Ingredients are listed by weight, from most to least, to help give you an idea of how specific ingredients compare with others in proportion.

The ingredient label is vital to people allergic to certain foods and/or additives. To help these people avoid problem ingredients, the ingredient list must include the following, when appropriate:

- FDA-certified color additives, such as FD&C Blue No. 1, by name.
- Sources of protein hydrolysates, which are used in many foods as flavors and flavor enhancers.
- Declaration of caseinate as a milk derivative in the ingredient list of foods that claim to be nondairy, such as coffee whiteners.

If you or your child has a food allergy or sensitivity, it is essential to identify what is safe to eat by searching the listed ingredients on a packaged food label. Specific questions about products should be directed to the food manufacturer. Most manufacturers offer a toll-free phone number that you can use to get specific questions answered.

Tips on the Food Label

It is important to use the food label for a number of reasons. It takes some practice, but once you begin to make reading the label a habit, it is hard not to use it. Keep these tips in mind when reading food labels:

- Read the serving size. The FDA requires that serving sizes reflect amounts customarily consumed for a food item and mandates that all like products use the same serving size. Remember also that all of the information pertains to that serving size.
- Determine the total calories per serving. To get a general idea of fat, take a look at how many of those calories per serving are coming from fat. Remember that there are only three nutrients that make up calories in food: fat, carbohydrate, and protein. So what is not fat is coming from protein and/or carbohydrate.
- Take a look at total fat content, but remember that it is also important to look at what type of fat is in the product. Determine the ratio of saturated fat to unsaturated fat or, if provided, the ratio of saturated fat to polyunsaturated fat to monounsaturated fat. Your daily accumulated ratio should consist of no more than 33 percent from saturated fat.

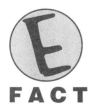

FACT

Food labels are changing all the time. To keep up with the latest information, check out the FDA's Web site at ✎*www.fda.gov* or use their toll-free number, ✆1-888-INFO-FDA.

- Determine whether your cholesterol intake is less than the budgeted 300 mg per day, and check to see if you have balanced out your day to fit the food in.

- Determine whether your sodium intake is less than the budgeted 2,400 mg per day, and check to see if you have balanced out your day to fit the food in.
- Determine total carbohydrates, and check to see how much of the total is coming from sugar, fiber, and complex carbohydrates. Whenever possible, choose foods that are higher in fiber and complex carbohydrates and lower in sugar.
- Don't overlook your vitamins and minerals. If you are choosing orange juice, for example, choose the one highest in vitamin C and the one that has been fortified with calcium. Pack in extra nutrition whenever you can!

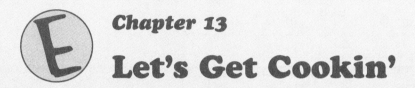

Chapter 13

Let's Get Cookin'

Cooking can be fun, delicious, and healthy. Making sure you have your kitchen stocked appropriately and learning to make some easy substitutions can help you convert most of your favorite recipes to healthier ones that can be a perfect match for your healthy lifestyle.

Stocking a Healthy Kitchen

Keeping a well-stocked kitchen can make it easier to prepare quick and healthy meals. It is helpful to stock your kitchen with a variety of basic foods. It is best to buy fresh ingredients as you need them.

Make sure to have the following on your kitchen shelf:

Brown rice and/or couscous	Brown sugar
Pasta	Honey
Bulgur or barley	Cornstarch
Beans (dried or canned)	Baking powder and baking soda
Fat-free refried beans	Vinegar
Reduced-fat condensed cream soups (a variety)	Ketchup, mustard, light mayonnaise, and relish
Chicken or beef broth	Reduced-fat salad dressings
Salsa or picante sauce	Canned tuna or salmon (packed in water)
Pasta sauce	Peanut butter
Vegetable cooking spray	Ready-to-eat whole-grain cereals
Vegetable oil, such as olive oil	Oatmeal
Herbs and spices	Baking potatoes and/or yams
Flour	Dried fruit, such as apricots and raisins
Sugar	Bread crumbs

Try to have the following in your refrigerator:

Fresh fruit (variety)	Parmesan cheese
Fresh vegetables (variety)	Low-fat margarine or butter spray
100 percent fruit or vegetable juices	Eggs or egg substitute
Onions	Low-fat sliced cheese
Tortillas	Reduced-fat deli meat, such as turkey breast
Fat-free milk	Bottled lemon juice
Low-fat yogurt	Light soy sauce and teriyaki sauce
Low-fat cottage cheese	Fresh garlic

Try to have the following in your freezer:	
Frozen vegetables	Lean meats (chicken breasts, lean beef, pork loin chops)
Frozen chopped onions	Fish
Shredded low-fat cheese, variety of flavors	Frozen yogurt, sherbet, or sorbet; frozen juice bars

Once you have your kitchen stocked, it is time to turn those ingredients into wholesome, nourishing meals the whole family will love.

One large part of your kitchen stock will probably be meat, poultry, and fish. These foods can contribute a huge part of your fat content for the day, so it is important to choose cuts carefully. Certain cuts of meat, poultry, and fish are leaner than others. Look for these examples when stocking your kitchen:

Healthy meat, poultry, and fish stock	
Beef:	Choose USDA Select or Choice grades of lean beef trimmed of fat such as round, sirloin, flank steak, eye of round, top round steak, top loin steak, tenderloin, roast (rib, chuck, rump), steak (porterhouse, T-bone, cube), ground round
Poultry:	Chicken or turkey (white meat, no skin), Cornish hen (no skin)
Pork:	Canadian bacon, tenderloin, center loin chop
Lamb:	Roast, chop, leg
Veal:	Lean chop, roast
Fish:	Fresh or frozen cod, flounder, haddock, halibut, trout, fresh tuna, tuna canned in water, fresh salmon, salmon canned in water, catfish, canned sardines
Shellfish:	Clams, crab, lobster, scallops, shrimp, imitation shellfish, oysters

Substituting extra-lean ground beef, ground round, or ground turkey for regular ground beef will reduce fat content by 7 to 9 grams per ounce. That's a fat savings of 63 to 144 grams of fat in one pound of ground meat. Family favorites like Sloppy Joes, tacos, hamburgers, chili, spaghetti sauce, and meatloaf taste just as satisfying without all the saturated fat. To keep chicken, pork, or fish moist, poach it in heavy aluminum foil with herbs, onions, your favorite vegetables, and other flavorings. Secure the package well, and bake or grill.

Recipe Modification: Getting Started

Making a few easy substitutions and using healthful cooking techniques can help you rejuvenate your favorite family recipes. There is no single way to change a recipe, but making small changes here and there can make big differences nutritionally.

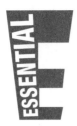

Just as important as having the right ingredients is having the correct utensils for cooking healthier. Get a good quality set of nonstick skillets, baking pans, and saucepans so you can sauté and bake without having to add extra fat.

You may have to use less of an ingredient, substitute one ingredient for another, take an ingredient out completely, or add a new ingredient. The result of each change may be just a little bit different, but that is all right. Substituting ingredients and making over a recipe may take some trial and error, but the result will make the effort worth it.

Use these steps to help you modify recipes:

1. Start by taking a look at the ingredients in the recipe and deciding which can be changed or modified to fit your nutritional goal, such as low fat, low sodium, or low sugar. Some ingredients have functional properties within the recipe, so be careful of what you change.
2. For easy substitutions, you can try substituting modified foods such as egg substitutes, reduced-fat cheese, reduced-fat sour cream, and sodium-reduced broth or soups.
3. Think about the ingredient you are going to replace. If it is salt, that is what may give flavor to the dish, so be sure to replace it with some herbs and spices. To add a little more fiber and cut some fat, you can substitute whole-wheat noodles for egg noodles.
4. Decide which ingredients you can eliminate altogether without altering the flavor or appearance of the dish.
5. Decide what ingredients you can add to the recipe to add nutritional value, such as adding wheat germ to casseroles or shredded carrots to lasagna. Both will go unnoticed but will add extra nutrition to the dish.

6. Make changes to your recipe gradually. Just make one or two ingredient changes the first time you modify it to see what the results are. If those few changes work well, try a few more the next time.

7. Modifying the method in which you prepare the dish can make big changes. Simple changes such as skimming the fat that collects on stew, rinsing ground meat after browning it, skipping the salt and oil in cooking water, or oven-baking chicken instead of frying it can all

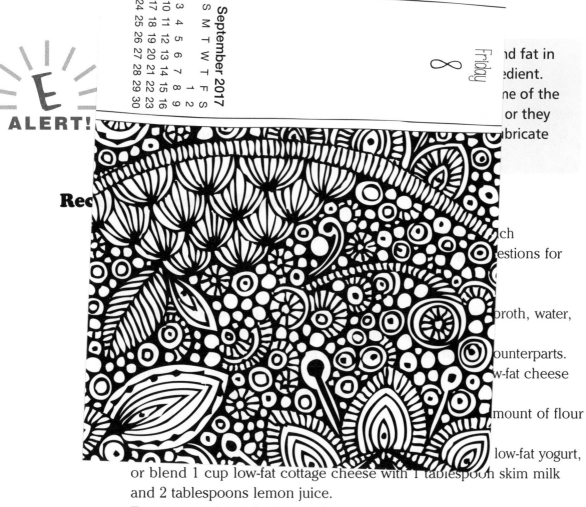

September 2017

S	M	T	W	T	F	S
					1	2
3	4	5	6	7	8	9
10	11	12	13	14	15	16
17	18	19	20	21	22	23
24	25	26	27	28	29	30

Friday

8

...d fat in
...edient.
...ne of the
...or they
...ubricate

E ALERT!

Rec...

...ch
...estions for

...broth, water,

...ounterparts.
...w-fat cheese

...mount of flour

...low-fat yogurt, or blend 1 cup low-fat cottage cheese with 1 tablespoon skim milk and 2 tablespoons lemon juice.

• For mayonnaise, substitute reduced-fat or fat-free versions, or use low-fat or fat-free plain yogurt.

• Because reduced-fat margarines are diluted with water, they should not be substituted for their full-fat counterparts one-to-one. To compensate for the extra water, substitute three-quarters as much of the light product for the full-fat margarine.

- Replace ricotta cheese with a lower-fat version or with 1 percent cottage cheese.
- Trim all visible fat and skin from meat before cooking.
- Replace a quarter to a half of the ground meat in casseroles or sauces with cooked brown rice, bulgur, couscous, dried beans, or tofu to decrease fat and increase fiber.
- Use puréed cooked vegetables instead of cream, egg yolks, or roux to thicken sauces and soups.

Not only can you modify your main meal dishes, but modifying your baked goods can also lead to enjoying healthier treats.

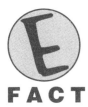

FACT

If sugar is the primary sweetener in your recipe that is not baked, scale down by 25 percent. For example, instead of 1 cup of sugar, use ¾ cup. Try adding a pinch of cinnamon, nutmeg, or allspice to increase the sweetness without adding extra calories.

Holiday Baking Tips

The holidays are the season for all kinds of goodies. Whether it's pumpkin pie, chocolate cake, or chocolate chip cookies, there are always plenty of sweet treats to choose from. Regardless of whether you are a baker, you may take to the kitchen at this time of year. The most popular holiday treats are usually quite high in fat, sugar, and calories. But you don't have to give up your favorite sweet treats if you modify your recipes to healthier versions. Here are just a few ideas:

- Substitute graham-cracker crusts for the traditional flour crusts on pies.
- Consider making apple, peach, or berry cobblers instead of a traditional pie; the dough used to make the cobbler is much lower in fat!
- For fat in baked goods such as pumpkin bread, banana bread, or

brownies, use an equivalent amount of applesauce as a substitute for most (or even all!) of the oil.

- Use nonfat condensed milk when a recipe calls for condensed milk, or use skim milk in place of whole milk.
- For filled cookies, use chopped dates or 100 percent fruit spread rather than jelly.
- If the recipe calls for nuts or coconut, reduce the amount and try toasting to enhance the flavor.
- To cut down on saturated fat content, use vegetable oils instead of margarine, butter, or lard in your recipes.
- Substitute half of the fat in a chocolate cake recipe with an equal amount of puréed prunes or low-fat mayonnaise.
- Increase fiber in baked goods by using whole-wheat flour for at least half of the all-purpose white flour.
- Use equal portions of evaporated milk as a substitute for heavy cream.
- Instead of spreading frosting on brownies or cakes, sprinkle powdered sugar on top or use a low-fat or fat-free whipped topping as frosting.
- If you decide to cook with artificial sweeteners, use a saccharin-based product. Aspartame breaks down and loses much of its sweetness when heated.
- If the recipe calls for baking chocolate, try cocoa instead. Replace one ounce of baking chocolate with 3 tablespoons cocoa powder plus 1 tablespoon vegetable oil.
- Since egg yolks, not egg whites, contain fat and cholesterol, use two egg whites or ¼ cup egg substitute for one whole egg.

Cooking Methods

The way you prepare your meal can make a big difference in the total fat, saturated fat, and cholesterol content. With simple changes to your cooking methods, you can cook leaner and still have great-tasting dishes. When deciding on a healthier cooking method, it is essential to understand key cooking methods and what they mean.

Most lower-fat cooking methods include braising, broiling, grilling, pan-broiling, poaching, roasting, simmering, steaming, stewing, and stir-frying.

Table 13-1 Cooking Methods	
Cooking Method	**Definition**
Braise	to simmer in a covered pot over low heat in a small amount of liquid such as water, broth, or fruit juice.
Broil	to cook with direct heat, usually under a heating element in the oven.
Fry	to cook food directly in hot oil.
Grill	to cook with direct heat over hot coals.
Pan-broil	to cook uncovered in a preheated, nonstick skillet without added oil or water.
Poach	to cook gently in liquid, just below the boiling point when the liquid is just beginning to show movement
Roast	to cook with dry heat in the oven.
Sauté	to cook quickly in a small amount of fat, stirring often so the food browns evenly.
Simmer	to cook slowly in liquid, just below boiling; usually done after reducing heat from a boil.
Steam	to cook with steam heat over (not in) boiling water.
Stew	to cook in enough liquid to cover food, such as water, broth, or stock, for a long period of time in a tightly covered pot over low heat.
Stir-fry	to cook small pieces of meat, poultry, fish, tofu, and/or vegetables in a very small amount of oil over very high heat, stirring often as it cooks.

Time-Saving Cooking Guidelines

Preparing a week's or more worth of meals at one time can help you eat healthy while saving time. Bulk cooking may make for a pretty busy weekend, but the payoff is a week or more of super easy and healthy dinners and more time for you during the week. A bulk cooking system is designed chiefly for main dishes, the most time-consuming part of a meal. Of course, they should be combined with vegetables, salad, and other healthy side dishes. Once you cook meals ahead, simply place them in freezer bags or airtight containers and freeze them. When you need a meal, it is as simple as taking it out of the freezer. Many foods freeze perfectly, especially soups, stews, spaghetti sauces, and chili. Let the food cool before you place it in the freezer, and be sure your freezer temperature is properly regulated (0 degrees or lower). Be careful not to stuff the freezer to the brim so air has room to circulate.

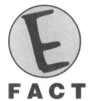

FACT

Try cooking rice, couscous, and other grains with herbs, fat-free broth, or juice instead of adding fat. Don't rinse rice when it is done cooking because you will wash away some of the vitamins, especially B vitamins.

Label your containers with contents and a date so you know what to use first and which dishes will keep for how long. As a rule of thumb, stews and casseroles will generally keep well for up to three months, while sauces will keep even longer. If you store frozen foods longer than what is recommended, they will generally still be safe to eat but the taste and texture may be compromised.

If you don't have the time to make so many meals at one time, try cooking a double batch of whatever meal you are making and freeze it for another meal the following week. Another time-saving tip is to use cooking methods such as grilling that make cooking and clean-up much easier.

Healthy Grilling

Grilling is a great way to get outside and do your cooking at the same time. It is quick as well as a great way to cook low-fat because you don't need to add any fat. Grilling does have a downside. Recent research has indicated that potential carcinogens (or substances that can cause cancer) are present in grilled foods. Fat that drips from the food onto the flames tends to create smoke that contains polycyclic aromatic hydrocarbons. These chemicals in the smoke can be potential carcinogens. The blackened parts of meat may also contain carcinogens. Just because grilled foods may contain some carcinogens does not mean that people who eat grilled food are going to develop cancer or that you should stop grilling. It is a smart idea nonetheless to reduce your exposure to carcinogens as much as possible. If you love to grill, follow these tips to help reduce your risk of exposure to possible carcinogens:

- To reduce grilling time, microwave or cook foods first that take a long time to cook on a grill. For example, cook ribs on low heat in the slow cooker or oven until cooked and then just put on the grill to baste with your favorite sauce.
- Use low or medium heat on the grill to avoid flames that shoot up and char the meat.
- Use leaner cuts of meat and marinades with little fat to avoid fat dripping on to the coals and causing flare-ups, smoke, and charring.
- Add glazes, sauces, or marinades only during the last few minutes on the grill; the sugar in the sauce causes flare-ups and increased smoke.
- Avoid eating the blackened parts of meat or other grilled foods.

Using Herbs and Spices

You need to keep some basic herbs and spices on hand to be prepared for any recipe. Using herbs and spices in your recipes offers a flavor advantage as you attempt to trim fat and sodium from your diet. Spices come from the bark, buds, fruit, roots, seeds, or stems of plants and trees. They are usually dried. Herbs, on the other hand, are the fragrant leaves of plants. Some plants supply both spices and herbs.

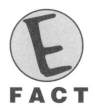
FACT

It is best to store dry herbs and spices in tightly covered containers and keep them in a cool, dry, dark place. Avoid storing them in the refrigerator, near a window, or above the stove. The atmosphere in some of these areas can destroy the flavor.

Herbs and spices lose their potency over time. As a rule of thumb, most whole herbs and spices retain their flavor for about one year. Dried and ground versions are best when used within six months. Before adding dried herbs to your recipe or dish, crush them between the palms of your hands to release their flavor. As a general rule for most herbs,

1 teaspoon of dried herb can be substituted for 1 tablespoon of chopped fresh herb. This is only a general guideline, so you should make sure to take your own tastes into consideration when selecting pantry basics.

Whether you are using fresh or dry seasonings, be sure to use them carefully—a little can go a long way. You can experiment with all types of combinations of herbs and spices to make up your own blends. Flavors will become more concentrated the longer the seasoning mixture is on the meat. In recipes that require a long cooking time, such as soups, stews, and sauces, add herbs and spices toward the end of cooking so their flavor won't cook out.

Herbs such as basil, bay leaf, oregano, or rosemary add distinctive flavors and color to meat, vegetables, and salads. Spices such as cinnamon, ginger, and nutmeg enhance the sweet taste of foods. Seasoning blends such as chili powder and curry powder provide complex flavors. If you are just starting to use herbs and spices, go slowly. Try one new spice at a time, and soon you'll love the new flavors.

Some basic herbs and spices for stocking your pantry include the following:

Allspice, ground and whole	Fennel seeds	Peppercorns, dried black
Arrowroot starch	Five-spice powder	Poppy seeds
Basil	Garlic powder	Rosemary, dried
Bay leaves	Ginger, ground	Sage, dried
Chili powder	Marjoram, dried	Salt, table and Kosher
Cinnamon, ground and sticks	Mint, dried	Sesame seeds
Cloves, ground and whole	Mustard, dried ground	Tarragon, dried
Coriander, ground	Nutmeg	Thyme, ground and dried
Cream of tartar	Onion powder	Turmeric
Cumin, ground	Oregano, dried	Vanilla extract
Curry powder	Paprika, Hungarian sweet	
Dill weed	Pepper, cayenne, dried red flakes	

A rub is a mixture of herbs and/or spices that is pressed onto the surface of meat before cooking. Rubs are commonly used on lean meats, poultry, and fish. Rubs can add lots of flavor to your meal without having to add fat or other higher-sodium marinades. Try some of these rub combinations for starters:

- **Citrus rub:** grated lemon, orange, or lime peel with minced garlic and black pepper.
- **Pork rub:** brown sugar, garlic powder, chili powder, black pepper, oregano, salt.
- **Italian rub:** oregano, basil, rosemary, minced Italian parsley, and garlic.

Herbs have recently received much attention for their possible medicinal benefits. Herbs and plants have a chemical structure and, like any chemical, can have some effect in the body. It is still uncertain how and which herbs may provide medical benefits as well as in what quantities. Begin to use herbs in cooking to help enhance flavor, and you can possibly provide a health benefit as well.

Finding a Good Cookbook

The following books and Web sites can help get your library started:

- *The All New Good Housekeeping Cookbook,* edited by Susan Westmoreland (Hearst Books)
- *American Heart Association Cookbook* (Random House, Inc.)
- *American Heart Association Meals in Minutes Cookbook* (Clarkson Potter Publishers)
- *Better Homes and Gardens New Cookbook* (Meredith Books, Inc.)
- *Vegetarian Times Complete Cookbook,* by Lucy Moll and *Vegetarian Times* editors (Hungry Minds, Inc.)
- *www.bhg.com*
- *www.cookinglight.com/cooking*
- *www.foodfit.com*
- *www.joyofcooking.com*
- *www.mealsforyou.com*

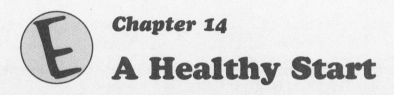

Chapter 14

A Healthy Start

Following sound nutrition guidelines can help take the guesswork out of the how, what, and whys of feeding your child throughout the infant and toddler years. The key for children is to provide proper nutrition and energy intake to support proper growth and development. Feeding your child can take time, patience, and plenty of creativity.

Breast Milk vs. Formula

One of the very first decisions new parents make, even before the baby is born, is how to feed their infant. Many health experts agree that breastfeeding is the ideal way, for optimum nutrition. Specifically, the American Dietetic Association (ADA) recommends that babies be breastfed exclusively for the first six months and then breastfed with complementary foods for at least twelve months. For those women not able to breastfeed or who choose not to, today's infant formulas provide a good nutritious alternative. Most are manufactured to be easy for babies to digest and to provide all the nutrition an infant needs.

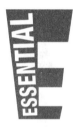

One advantage to breast milk is the protective substances it contains that help protect the baby from various infections. One such substance, called "colostrum," is a yellowish premilk substance secreted in the first few days after a woman delivers. It is believed to carry even more antibodies to help fight infection and is also rich in protein and zinc.

Advantages of Breastfeeding

Infants who are breastfed until they are satisfied, and infants who are fed a standard formula and whose mothers are in tune to their cues of hunger and satiety, will generally adjust their own intake to meet their calorie needs. There can be many advantages to breastfeeding your newborn baby. Breast milk seems to be the perfect form of nutrition for a human baby's delicate digestive system. All of breast milk's components, including lactose, protein (whey and casein), and fat, are easily digested by a newborn's immature system. Commercial formulas attempt to reproduce these ingredients and are coming quite close, though the exact combination cannot be duplicated. Breast milk contains the vitamins and minerals that a newborn requires, and breastfed babies supposedly have fewer allergies later in life.

Since breast milk is easily and quickly digested, breastfed babies sometimes tend to eat more often than formula-fed babies. This can be tiring for Mom, but it does not take long for these babies to feed less frequently and to sleep through the night. Breastfeeding can require quite a bit of commitment from a mother, especially for new moms who go back to work outside of the home or who are separated from their babies from time to time for other reasons. In these cases, a breast pump may be used to collect breast milk. Some mothers are able to breastfeed most of the time and use bottle feedings at other times.

Advantages of Formula Feeding

There can also be advantages to formula-feeding your newborn baby. Commercially prepared infant formulas can be a nutritious and more convenient alternative to breastfeeding, and they even contain iron.

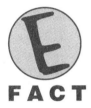

FACT

Iron-fortified infant formulas have actually been credited for the declining incidence of anemia in infants. For this reason, the American Academy of Pediatrics highly recommends that mothers who are not breastfeeding use an iron-fortified infant formula.

Today's commercial formula products are manufactured under strict sterile conditions, and producers do attempt to duplicate the ingredients found in breast milk. It would be virtually impossible for a mother to create a formula at home with the same complex combination of proteins, sugars, fats, vitamins, and minerals that a baby needs and that are present in commercial formulas. If you do not breastfeed your baby, use only a commercially prepared formula.

Some women feel that bottle-feeding their infant gives them a little more freedom and that other members of the family can be more active in the feeding and caring of the infant. Just as breastfeeding has its own unique demands, so does bottle-feeding. The main demands of bottle-feeding are organization and preparation. You need to make sure to have enough formula on hand, and bottles must be prepared very carefully. The bottles and nipples must be kept sanitary and ready when you need them.

The baby's bottle should be warmed just slightly before feeding. Never heat a bottle of formula in a microwave! The formula can heat unevenly and leave hot spots, which can burn a baby's mouth. A microwave can also heat the formula too much, making it too hot for an infant's mouth. The best way is to heat water in the microwave, take the water out, and then heat the bottle in the water. Always test the formula to make sure it is not too hot.

Bottle-feeding can be more costly. The decision to breastfeed or bottle-feed your baby should be based on your comfort level with breastfeeding—as well as on your lifestyle.

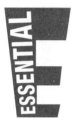

If bottles are left out of the refrigerator for longer than one hour or the baby doesn't finish a bottle, they should be discarded. Prepared formula bottles should be stored in the refrigerator for no longer than twenty-four hours.

Starting Solid Foods

Starting your baby on solid foods is the beginning of lifelong eating habits that will contribute to his or her overall health. The American Academy of Pediatrics recommends feeding your child only breast milk or formula for the first four to six months of life. After that, a combination of solid foods and breast milk or formula should be given until your baby is at least a year old. After babies reach six months, their nutritional needs are more than breast milk or formula can provide alone.

What Age to Start

Be cautious of starting babies on solid food too soon. Starting solid foods too early can cause babies to develop food allergies. This is because their intestinal tracts and immune systems are not yet fully developed; introducing solid foods at this time can be too much for them to handle. Starting a baby on solid foods too soon, before four to six months, can also cause overfeeding since they cannot yet offer you signals as to when they are full. There is also the danger of a baby's being unable to chew or swallow correctly before this age.

At four to six months, breast milk or formula is the only food that your baby needs, but you can still begin to familiarize your baby with the feel of a spoon and begin to introduce solid foods. Iron-fortified rice cereal is the least allergenic and is recommended as the first type of solid food that should be introduced. You can mix 1 tablespoon of rice cereal with breast milk, formula, or water and feed it to the baby with a spoon (not a bottle). Offer cereal two to three times per day.

After cereal has passed the test and the baby is about five to six months old, you can move on puréed fruit and vegetables. Continue to give breast milk or formula and iron-fortified cereal each day. Offer 1 to 2 tablespoons of strained vegetables or fruit two to three times per day. Offer one new food every three to four days, and watch for signs of intolerance.

By age six to eight months, a baby's digestive tract is more mature, and you can begin to introduce more types of foods. While continuing to give breast milk or formula, increase iron-fortified cereal to 4 tablespoons or more daily. Increase strained vegetables to 2 tablespoons or more per day, and increase strained fruits to 2 tablespoons or more per day. You can now start to offer plain strained meats such as chicken, beef, turkey, veal, lamb, or egg yolks (no egg whites as there is a high chance of allergic reactions in infants younger than twelve months old). Offer ½ to 1 tablespoon one to two times daily. You can also begin to offer 2 to 4 ounces of 100 percent fruit juices. Start by mixing one part juice with two parts water, and offer it in a cup.

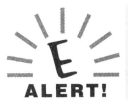

ALERT!

If using commercially prepared baby food, do not use vegetables with meat because they have little meat and less protein and iron than jars with plain meat. If your baby doesn't like plain meat, mix it with a vegetable that they already like as you offer it.

At this age you can also start to offer soft table foods and finger foods. Begin with soft, bite-size pieces of food, such as unsweetened dry cereals, crackers, and soft breads. Never give these types of foods to children unless you are with them in case of choking.

At eight to nine months, continue with the breast milk or formula and iron-fortified cereal. Begin trying junior foods (half jar) or mashed and chopped table foods such as meat, poultry, potato, or well-cooked pieces of vegetable. Chopped canned fruit can replace strained fruit (be sure fruit is canned in light syrup or its own juices). Begin to also offer one to two small servings of bread, crackers, solid cereals, toast, or zwieback. Offer small servings of cottage cheese, plain yogurt, and soft cheeses. At this point you can increase the amount of food your baby is eating according to the baby's appetite.

From ten to twelve months, continue with breast milk or formula and iron-fortified cereals (4 tablespoons or more per day). At this point you can add cooked, cut-up pieces of vegetables, soft fruits, and tender meats. Casseroles with pasta or rice can be introduced. Again, increase the amount of food according to the baby's appetite. It is important to offer a variety of foods to encourage good eating habits later.

After the First Year

After twelve months of age, you can give your baby homogenized whole cow's milk. Do not use 2 percent, low-fat, or skim milk until your child is two or three years old.

If using soy milk after your child is a year old, keep in mind that it is low in fat. A toddler soy formula may be a better alternative, or you can make up for the reduced fat intake from milk in other areas of your child's diet.

Keep in mind that your baby's appetite may decrease and become pickier over the next few years as his or her growth rate slows.

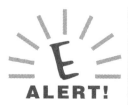

ALERT!

Avoid putting your baby down for a nap or to sleep with a bottle of formula or juice, which allows sugar to collect in the baby's mouth and can lead to cavities. Also, do not give carbonated or caffeinated drinks, candy, or other foods that your baby may choke on, such as grapes, hot dogs, or thick and sticky foods like peanut butter.

Growth Charts

The National Center for Health Statistics has developed growth charts that are used to compare a child's measurements with those of other children the same age. By plotting a child's measurements on these charts, doctors are able to compare individual growth patterns with data collected on thousands of U.S. children. This helps to determine whether a child's growth is normal compared with others the same age. Boys and girls are plotted on different charts because of their difference in growth rates and patterns. There are two sets of standard charts for both boys and girls: one for infants aged newborn to thirty-six months and another for children ages two to twenty years. The charts are a series of percentile curves that show the distribution of growth measurements of children from across the country.

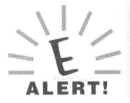
ALERT!

Only those measurements obtained in your child's doctor's office or taken by another health professional should be plotted. Many times home measurements are inaccurate and inconsistent, which can lead to incorrect data and unnecessary concern.

During your child's routine visits to the doctor, certain measurements will be taken and recorded in the child's medical record. With an older child, a doctor may plot up to four numbers on the growth chart: height for age, weight for age, weight for height, and a recent addition, body mass index (BMI). Infants are usually measured for length for age, weight for age, weight for length, and head circumference for age.

A growth chart contains seven curves that all follow the same standard pattern. Each curve represents a different percentile: the fifth, tenth, twenty-fifth, fiftieth, seventy-fifth, ninetieth, and ninety-fifth. The fiftieth percentile represents the average value for age. A child's continued growth measurements are plotted among the percentile curves. For example, an infant whose head circumference falls in the ninetieth percentile is plotted on the second curve from the top of the chart. Being in the ninetieth percentile means the child's head measurement is greater than or equal to the measurements of 90 percent of children in the country in the same age category. The remaining 10 percent of children that age have greater head measurements. Just because a child has a high or low reading does not always mean there is a problem.

Generally, if a measurement exceeds the ninety-fifth percentile, or if it crosses two percentile curves (for example, climbing from the forty-fifth to the seventy-fifth percentile, thereby crossing the fiftieth and seventy-fifth percentile curves), there may be some cause for concern.

If a measurement falls below the fifth percentile, or if it crosses two percentile curves (for example, dropping from the fiftieth to the twentieth percentile), there may be some cause for concern. The doctor may consider health problems affecting the child's normal growth pattern.

Growth charts can be valuable tools, but it is important not to focus too much on any one reading. When growth chart readings are examined over time, they reveal a pattern of development. It is the pattern that tells you whether a child is growing properly in relation to other children the same age. The pattern also shows how the child is progressing from measurement to measurement. This is a much more useful indicator of a child's development than any single measurement.

Food Allergies

It is important to be aware of food allergies, especially if your child may be at risk for developing a food allergy. Children can be at higher risk if they have an allergy to any type of food or formula or if they have other family members with food allergies. If you are not breastfeeding, or if you need to supplement, consider using a hypoallergenic infant formula. If you are breastfeeding, avoid milk, eggs, fish, peanuts, and tree nuts in your diet.

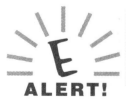

Soy formulas and goat's milk may not be good alternatives to formula because many infants who are allergic to cow's milk may also be allergic to soy.

If your child is at high risk of developing food allergies, delay offering solid food until the child is at least six months old. At this time you can begin an iron-fortified infant cereal while continuing to breastfeed. Start with rice and oat cereals, and introduce wheat cereals later on. Next try introducing vegetables, but avoid legumes (dried beans and peas) at first. Next would come noncitrus fruits and juices. Meat and protein-type foods can be added when the child reaches eight to nine months.

Avoid egg whites, cow's milk, wheat, and citrus fruits and juices until your infant is at least one year old. Peanuts (including peanut butter) and shellfish should also be avoided until your child is at least two to three years old.

Be careful of feeding your child mixed-ingredient foods unless you are sure that he or she is not allergic to any of the individual ingredients. Also, avoid adding any seasonings to the food until your child is a bit older.

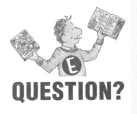

QUESTION?

Will avoiding certain foods during pregnancy prevent a baby from developing food allergies?
No concrete scientific evidence proves that restricting certain foods during pregnancy will prevent a baby from developing a food allergy. In fact, it is not recommended for women to restrict their diets while pregnant. Mothers who restrict their diets during pregnancy often have a lower birth-weight baby.

When you offer a new food, feed it to the child for several days in a row before you offer another new one. This makes it easier to detect food allergies. Symptoms of food allergies can include diarrhea, vomiting, nausea, swelling around the mouth or throat, coughing, difficulty breathing, wheezing, hives, or a rash. Symptoms usually develop fairly quickly after the child eats a specific food, sometimes within minutes to hours. More common than food allergies are intolerances to certain foods, which can also cause vomiting, diarrhea, spitting up, and skin rashes. If you suspect a food allergy in your child, keep a food diary for a few weeks and record what foods your child has been eating, especially newly introduced foods, and when the symptoms developed. That may help you to figure out exactly what food is causing the allergic reaction. Most kids outgrow food allergies; however, allergies to peanuts and tree nuts are seldom outgrown.

Your doctor should decide if and when you can begin reintroducing foods that have caused allergic actions in the past.

Toddlers and Preschoolers

Children in their toddler and preschool year are very impressionable, which makes it the perfect time to help them form good eating habits. Children are never too young to establish a foundation of good nutrition and healthy eating habits.

Toddlers and preschoolers grow at a slower rate than infants. They need enough energy or calories to fuel their active play and their various stages of growth, but they do not need adult-size portions. Large portions can overwhelm their small appetites and are too big for their small stomachs. Servings for these children should be a quarter to a third the size of an adult portion. Children do not need as much food as an adult. They really only need enough to satisfy their hunger, so listen to their cues. When children say they are done, remove the food or let them leave the table.

Make mealtime enjoyable and pleasant for you and your child and not a source of constant struggle. To help make sure your child eats well, do not allow him or her to drink too many beverages at meals—such as milk, juice, or water—so that they are not hungry for solid foods. Refrain from forcing your child to eat when he or she is not hungry or from forcing unwanted foods. Also avoid giving large amounts of sweet desserts, soft drinks, fruit-flavored drinks, sugarcoated cereals, chips, or candy. These foods have little to no nutritional value and will fill a child up quickly, leaving little room for more nutritious foods.

The following tips can make mealtime more pleasant for both you and your child:

- Plan a quiet time before meals and snacks. Children tend to eat better if they are relaxed.
- Encourage children to sit at the table when they eat, and give them plenty of time to eat their meal.
- Even if you are not eating with your children, sit at the table with

them. Young children should be supervised while they eat to aid in encouragement and in case of choking.

- Don't use food as a reward or as a punishment. This can lead to unhealthy attitudes toward eating and food.
- Respect your children's food preferences, and let them choose or reject foods as adults or older children do.
- Get your children involved in preparing certain parts of the meal.
- Make every effort to make eating, and not watching television, the main focus of the family meal.
- Use child-size dishes and utensils that the child can handle with ease. Using too large a plate can be overwhelming.
- Offer foods with kid appeal. Younger children usually like plain, unmixed foods as well as finger-foods that making eating easier.
- Offer plenty of variety from each of the food groups. If your children don't like spinach, don't assume they don't like vegetables. Just offer another vegetable.

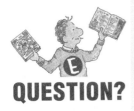

QUESTION?

Should I worry that my child is not getting enough to eat? Probably not. Children will generally eat when they are hungry and stop when they are full. Young children don't need a whole lot of food and will generally get what their body needs. If you are worried, speak to your pediatrician.

How Much Food Is Enough?

Children do better on an eating schedule. Even though you should offer the child three balanced meals a day, they will probably only eat one or two. Because children have a limited stomach capacity, it is best to feed them five to six small daily meals. Plan nutritious snacks as part of the day's meal schedule. Children's appetites change from day to day, which is completely normal. To help stimulate a good appetite, children should be active and spend time outside in the fresh air. Children will not eat well if they are tired. Schedule mealtimes and play times accordingly. It doesn't take much to satisfy a child's small appetite, so plan meals well.

If they snack right before a meal, their intake at that meal will not be as good. Children should not be given any food or drink within an hour and a half of a meal.

As long as a child is growing normally, he or she is getting enough calories. A child's food intake usually increases just before a growth spurt.

FIGURE 14-1
The Kids'
Food Pyramid
(for ages two
through six)

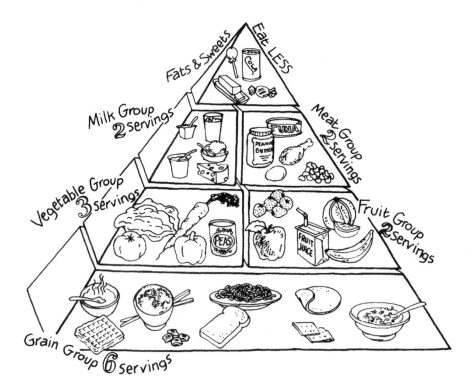

Food Jags

Food jags are periods when children refuse foods that they previously liked or when they repeatedly request a particular food at each meal. This behavior is commonly observed in toddlers and preschoolers between the ages of two to six. During these years, growth is slower and appetite tends to decrease. This can cause concern and frustration in parents who want to be sure the child is getting adequate nutrition. Children at this age are more interested in discovering the world around them than in the food they eat. Food jags can happen because the child is bored with the usual foods or is trying to discover a new independence.

The best way to handle a toddler's food jags is to remain low key. The more you focus on it, the longer the food jag may last. Being either too rigid or too accommodating will not help. Children cannot be forced to eat foods they do not want. Food preferences develop as a child is exposed to new foods in a calm, nonthreatening environment. Realize that this is a temporary situation and a normal part of the child's development. You still have control over what foods are offered to the child, so continue to offer a variety of foods and allow the child to make food choices from what is available. It is fine to offer the food they want again and again as long as other foods are offered to encourage variety. They will probably become bored with the same food and begin eating others that are offered. Offer their favorite foods as well as substitutions for the foods they refuse. Children will meet all of their nutritional needs over several days' time.

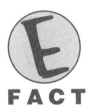

FACT

Toddlers control very few things in their environment. When a child discovers how upsetting it can be to a parent when they refuse to eat or demand the same food at meals, eating behavior can become a powerful tool for getting attention.

Continue to offer healthy and nutritious foods, and plan mealtimes appropriately. When a child sits down to eat, step back and allow the child to control what he or she eats. This will enable your child to develop healthy eating behaviors. If a child refuses entire food groups for more than two weeks, talk to a doctor or registered dietitian.

Trying New Foods

Getting your child to try a new food can be frustrating. Keep in mind that taste is not the only factor that is important in a child's food acceptance. Temperature of food is also important. Most toddlers will do best with lukewarm foods.

To help your child try new foods, try the following tips:

- Offer just one new food at a time. Let the child know if the taste is sweet, sour, or salty.
- Let children taste a very small amount at first to see if they like it.
- Tell children that if they don't like it, they don't have to swallow it.
- Many young children have to be offered a food several times before they accept it. If they don't accept it the first time, try again later.
- Be a role model. A caregiver who asks a child to drink milk or eat vegetables should be doing the same.
- When introducing a new food, seat the child with a sibling or friends who are good tasters and will eat the food.
- When serving a new food, serve it with one the child already likes.

The odor and presentation of food are also factors in whether the child will be open to trying a new food.

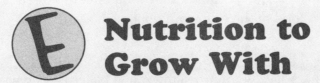

Chapter 15

Nutrition to Grow With

School-age children and teenagers are much more independent when it comes to making food choices. Children and young adults need a different type of guidance. No matter what their age, learning the importance of a healthy diet and a healthy weight is essential to good health and growing into a healthy adult.

Nutrition for School-Age Children

School-age children are no longer toddlers yet not quite teenagers. At this age they are beginning to eat away from home and make their own food choices more frequently. Children at this age grow at a rapid pace.

Children need the same nutrients as adults but in different amounts. Just as it is for adults, it is important for growing children to eat a variety of foods from each food group to ensure optimal intake of all vitamins and minerals.

A well-nourished and fit child is better able to learn and has more energy, stamina, and self-esteem. A healthy eating pattern along with regular exercise helps children to get fit. The calorie needs of school-age children vary greatly and depend on growth rate, activity level, and body size. All children need at least the lowest end of the serving range from each food group in the Food Guide Pyramid. Most school-age children need about 1,000 to 2,200 calories each day. **TABLE 15-1** gives the number of servings in each food group for this caloric intake.

Table 15-1 Number of Servings for Children Aged Six to Twelve	
Food Group	**Number of Servings***
Bread, Cereal, Rice, and Pasta	6–9
Vegetables	3–4
Fruit	2–3
Milk, Yogurt, and Cheese	2–3
Meat, Poultry, Fish, Dry Beans, Eggs, and Nuts	2–3 (about 5–6 ounces)

*Children may prefer smaller servings than those indicated in Chapter 3. Serving several smaller serving sizes can still add up to the total recommended number of servings for the day.

Eating at School

For school-age children, school meals can contribute significantly to overall daily dietary intake. Some children may bring their lunch from home, while others may participate in the school lunch program. The National School Lunch Program, regulated by the U.S. Department of

Agriculture (USDA), provides about a third of the RDA for students. Children from low-income families are eligible for free or reduced-price meals.

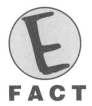

FACT

Children grow rapidly during these years—typically, they grow one to two feet in height and almost double their weight from six to twelve years of age.

School meals are planned to help moderate fat intake and offer more fiber through whole grains and fresh fruits. It is a smart idea to become familiar with the menu if your child participates in the school lunch program. If your child carries a lunch to school, pack lunches that are pleasing as well as fun to eat, healthy, safe, and nutritious. A well-balanced packed lunch might include a sandwich with whole wheat-bread and a lean, protein-rich filling, such as turkey, chicken, tuna, egg, cheese, or peanut butter; fresh fruit and/or vegetables; low-fat or fat-free milk; and graham crackers, Jell-O, or another simple low-fat dessert. Be aware of food safety measures when packing your child's lunch, such as keeping perishable foods well chilled.

Eating after School

School-age children primarily consume snacks after school. After-school snacks can be a nutritious way to make sure children get the energy and nutrients they need to properly fuel their bodies and to ensure proper growth and development. Snacking can be part of a healthy diet if snacks are chosen correctly. It is another opportunity to incorporate needed food groups into the child's daily diet.

Some speedy after-school snack ideas include the following:

- Bagel or English muffin pizza
- Shaker pudding. Pour 2 cups milk into a jar with a lid, add 1 small box instant pudding mix, and shake for one minute.
- Tortilla rollups. Roll a tortilla with shredded cheese, microwave until cheese is soft, and dip in salsa.

- Peanut butter on a mini bagel
- Cereal topped with fruit and milk
- Cheese and crackers
- Fruited yogurt topped with granola
- Cut-up vegetables dipped in low-fat ranch salad dressing
- Sunflower seeds
- Pretzels
- Banana pops. Peel a banana, dip it in yogurt, then crush in breakfast cereal or granola; freeze.
- Celery with low-fat cream cheese
- Peanut butter on graham crackers
- Fresh fruit (cut up and ready in a bowl, easy to grab and eat)
- Low-fat string cheese
- Breakfast bars
- Banana or apple topped with peanut butter
- Fruit shake-up. Put ½ cup low-fat yogurt and ½ cup cold fruit juice in an unbreakable, covered container. Shake it up and pour it in a cup.

The Dilemma of Overweight Children

The percentage of overweight children, aged six to seventeen years, has doubled in the United States since 1968. A National Health and Nutrition Examination Survey conducted by the National Center for Health Statistics from 1988 to 1994 found that one in five children in the United States was overweight. Studies also show that almost 70 percent of overweight kids aged ten to thirteen will be overweight or obese as adults.

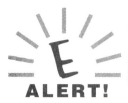

ALERT!

An increasing number of teenagers are also overweight, and, if no intervention is made, approximately 80 percent of them will stay overweight or become obese as adults.

Children and teens will probably experience psychological and emotional fallout from being overweight as youngsters. They may struggle with self-esteem, and they often become the object of teasing from other children. Overweight children are also put at risk for health problems. Studies show that overweight children tend to have higher levels of blood sugar, blood pressure, and blood fats.

Children can become overweight for a variety of reasons. The most common are genetic factors, lack of physical activity, unhealthy eating patterns, or a combination. In rare cases, a medical problem can cause a child to become overweight.

Assessing whether a child's weight put him or her in an overweight category can be difficult because children grow in erratic spurts. If you feel your child or teen may be overweight, consult your family physician. Your doctor may use growth charts, such as the ones discussed in Chapter 14, to determine if there is a problem.

Handling an Overweight Child

Children and teens should never be placed on a calorie-restricted diet to lose weight unless they are under the strict supervision of a doctor for medical reasons. Limiting what children or teens eat can be harmful to their health and can interfere with proper growth and development. It can also be psychologically stressful for a child. Helping the child to adopt healthy eating and exercise habits is more important than pounds lost. Behavior modification strategies have shown considerable success in effecting long-term weight loss. The best programs incorporate plenty of physical activity and healthy eating, including slowing the rate of eating, limiting the time and place of eating, and teaching problem-solving through exercises. The most effective treatments also involve parents.

To help your child achieve a healthy weight, try the following techniques:

- Seek the advice of a health-care professional, such as a registered dietitian or doctor. Keep in mind that adult approaches to weight loss are not fit for children.
- Give your children support, acceptance, and encouragement, no matter what their weight, and talk to them about their feelings. This

will help them carry a positive self-image, making weight loss more achievable.

- Starting in early childhood, teach children proper nutrition, selection of healthy low-fat snacks, and the importance of physical activity. Monitor the time they spend watching television or sitting at a computer.

- Make it a point to include good nutrition, and make exercise a family affair. Plan lower-fat meals for the entire family, have more nutritious snacks in the house, and plan family activities. This will help the child feel part of the family instead of isolated (not to mention that the whole family will benefit!).

- Beware of using food as a reward for a certain accomplishment, as a substitute for affection, or as a compensation for a disappointment. Use other avenues as rewards.

- Make sure your child's portions are a child's as opposed to an adult's size. Use smaller plates for children so you or the child is not tempted to fill up a large plate.

- Explain to children how to recognize when their body tells them that they are hungry or full.

- Stock your kitchen with low-fat and low-calorie snack foods so they are available when the child is hungry. Be aware of bringing high-fat, high-calorie foods into the house and having them within sight of the child.

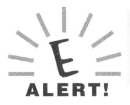
ALERT!

Although limiting fat intake may help prevent excess weight gain in children, it is not recommended to restrict fat intake in children who are younger than two.

- Instead of heavy snacking, make meals their primary source of calories.

- Do not encourage continued eating or cleaning their plates when children are truly no longer hungry.

- Avoid labeling foods as "good" or "bad." Instead, help your child to learn how to fit all types of food into a healthy eating pattern, and teach them how to eat foods in moderation. Even if your child has a few pounds to lose, he or she can still eat foods such as sweets in moderation. What counts is their diet as a whole.

- Make a family rule that eating is only allowed in the kitchen or dining room to keep kids from snacking on high-calorie foods while watching television. Children will most likely eat less with this rule in place.

Feeding Your Teen

By the time a child reaches the teen years, he or she has a major influence on food choices. Compared to when they were in their childhood years, teens are probably eating away from home more often than just at school. Teens understand the basics of good nutrition but many stray due to peer pressure, work and school schedules, the need to test independence, lack of discipline, lack of a good example at home, or obsessions with an unrealistic body weight. As with adults or children, the Food Guide Pyramid is also a guideline for teens. Because of an increased need for calories, teens need to increase their number of food group servings to meet their nutritional needs. Teenage boys from eleven to fourteen need about 2,500 calories per day, and boys aged fifteen to eighteen need about 2,800 calories. Refer to **TABLE 15-2** to find the appropriate number of servings for this caloric range.

Table 15-2 Number of Servings for Teenage Boys	
Food Group	**Number of Servings***
Bread, cereal, rice, and pasta	10–11
Vegetables	4–5
Fruit	3–4
Milk, yogurt, and cheese	3
Meat, poultry, fish, dry beans, eggs, and nuts	2–3 (about 6–7 ounces)

*Teens will probably eat servings more closely resembling the size of an adult serving.

On average, teenage girls need 2,200 calories per day from eleven to eighteen. See **TABLE 15-3** for the number of servings from each group girls in this category require.

Table 15-3	Number of Servings for Teenage Girls
Food Group	Number of Servings*
Bread, cereal, rice, and pasta	9
Vegetables	4
Fruit	3
Milk, yogurt, and cheese	3
Meat, poultry, fish, dry beans, eggs, and nuts	2 (about 6 ounces)

*Teens will eat servings more closely resembling the size of an adult serving.

Teens' Special Needs

Two nutrients typically come up short in a teen's diet: calcium and iron. This usually happens due to poor eating habits, poor food choices, or not eating enough. Calcium-rich foods are vital to ensure strong healthy bones. Even as teenagers reach their adult height, bones continue to grow stronger and denser. Almost half of your bone mass as an adult is formed during the teen years.

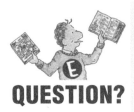

QUESTION?

What else can teens do for healthy bones?
Besides eating a diet rich in calcium including milk, cheese, yogurt, and calcium-fortified foods, teens should participate in weight-bearing physical activities. These may include running, tennis, soccer, dancing, volleyball, or inline skating. These types of activities trigger the formation of bone tissue. Also, they should go easy on soft-drinks, especially caffeinated ones, and avoid smoking.

Fatigue can be a sign of iron deficiency. When iron is in short supply, less oxygen is available to produce energy. Iron needs increase during the teen years. Girls need more iron to replace losses from their menstrual blood flow, and both boys and girls need more iron due to more muscle mass and greater blood supply. Iron comes from foods such as meat, poultry, seafood, legumes, enriched grains, and some vegetables.

It is important for teenagers to eat at least three meals per day to ensure they are consuming all needed nutrients. A meal skipped on occasion is not a concern, but skipping meals on a regular basis can mean missing out on essential nutrients.

Being physically active is just as essential to teenagers as it is to adults. One reason teens are not as active these days is too many sedentary activities, such as television; too many hours at the computer; and video games. Helping teens establish a lifelong habit of being physically active can help reduce their risk now for chronic health problems later in life. Keep in mind that you are a role model for your teen!

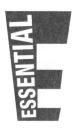

Boys and girls aged seven to ten need about 10 mg of iron daily. For girls during adolescence, aged eleven to eighteen years, the need jumps to 15 mg daily. For boys during adolescence, age eleven to eighteen years, the need jumps to 12 mg per day.

Eating Disorders

The teenage years can be difficult for both boys and girls. To most teens, their looks are extremely important, with the main focus usually being body image. Often, teens have unrealistic notions about the way their body should look. Boys usually put more emphasis on exercising, especially with weights. Teenage girls tend to diet as an approach to finding the perfect body. This usually involves some type of fad diet, and that can be very dangerous, especially during the adolescent years. Excessive concern about weight can also lead girls to engage in unhealthy behaviors, such as excessive exercise, self-induced vomiting, and the abuse of medications such as laxatives or diuretics.

Being obsessive about weight can result in various eating disorders. It is estimated that one million or more Americans suffer from some type of eating disorder. Eating disorders are more than a food problem and are linked to psychological problems.

Anorexia and Bulimia

Anorexia nervosa is a common eating disorder that usually begins at the age of fourteen or fifteen (but can occur at a younger age), with another peak in incidence in eighteen-year-olds. It is more common in adolescent girls, but it is also found in boys and its incidence has been increasing. Anorexia causes an overwhelming fear of being overweight and a drive to be thin, leading to self-induced starvation or a severe restriction of calories that can lead to being severely underweight. Anorexia is linked to menstrual irregularity, osteoporosis (brittle bone disease) in women, and a greater risk of early death in both men and women.

Bulimia is another eating disorder marked by a loss of control and binge eating, followed by purging behaviors. The person gorges on high-calorie foods and then intentionally vomits or uses laxatives or diuretics.

Signs to Watch For

Factors that you should look for if you suspect that your child has an eating disorder include the following:

- Low self-esteem
- Recent weight loss of 15 percent or more of normal body weight, with no medical reason
- A fear of gaining weight or of being overweight
- Purging behaviors (vomiting or using diuretics—water pills—or laxatives to lose weight)
- Having a distorted image of their body size or shape (for example, believing they are overweight even though they are at a healthy weight or even underweight)
- A preoccupation with thoughts of food, calories, and weight

- Restrictive eating patterns such as frequently skipping meals, fasting, or eliminating entire food groups
- Preference for eating alone
- For young women, amenorrhea (absence of menstrual cycles) or delayed onset of puberty
- Being underweight, with a body mass index that is below normal
- Exercising compulsively
- An extreme denial of possibility of eating disorder
- Withdrawal from friends and family
- Wearing bulky clothing to hide weight loss
- A recent or past event in their life that was very stressful

You should have your child seen by a physician as soon as possible if you think she or he might have an eating disorder. Eating disorders can cause extreme undernourishment and even death. The best treatment for eating disorders combines medical, psychological, and nutrition counseling.

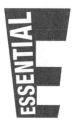

For more information on eating disorders, contact the National Eating Disorders Association at *www.nationaleatingdisorders.org* or the Renfrew Center at *www.renfrew.org*.

The College Years

By the time college rolls around, food choices are completely up to the young adult. College can be a time of rush, rush, rush and not having enough time or money for good eating habits. College dorm life is a particularly toxic food environment, with limited cafeteria food choices, vending machines, a general lack of nutritional consciousness, and the ease of getting deliverable foods like pizza. College life can bring on sloppy eating habits as well as a lack of exercise habits, not to mention some alcohol and partying. Along with all the other changes that college brings, changes in eating habits are sure to happen. It is not unusual for the college freshman to put on an extra 15 pounds during the first year at school.

Skipping Breakfast

One of the number-one mistakes college kids make is skipping breakfast. As we have discussed before, breakfast is the most important meal of the day. When you wake up in the morning, your body has gone for about eight hours with no food or fuel. Breakfast can be a bagel and juice in your room or on the way to class; whole-grain cereal, fat-free milk, and fruit in the dining hall; or even a hot meal. Breakfast can help get your brain and body ready for your hectic day and make you less likely to snack on high-fat, high-calorie foods between classes due to midmorning hunger attacks. Breakfast can also keep you more awake and alert for those early morning classes!

Campus Dining Halls

Campus dining halls are filled with both healthy and not-so-healthy foods. The key is learning what to choose.

At breakfast, stick with whole-grain cereals, bagels, toast, and other starches with low-fat toppings. Top your cereal with fresh fruit and top it off with fat-free milk. Choose low-fat yogurts for added calcium and egg whites or hard-boiled eggs for added protein. Avoid sugary cereals and higher-fat breakfast foods like doughnuts, Danish, bacon, sausage, or eggs fried in fat. Some of those may be quicker to prepare but are full of fat, sugar, and extra calories. These types of food will put on the pounds and not keep you satisfied as long.

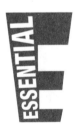

If you visit the salad bar, avoid too much fat and too many calories: use only a small amount of low-fat or fat-free salad dressing; avoid vegetable salads made with mayonnaise; use only a sprinkling of cheese, nuts, or seeds; use legumes such as garbanzo beans or kidney beans for added protein; and fill up your bowl with fresh, plain veggies.

At lunch, visit the deli section and choose a whole-wheat pita stuffed with plenty of veggies and some lean roast beef, turkey, or ham. Add some light mayonnaise or mustard. Tuna salad or chicken salad can be high in fat and calories because it's often made with too much mayonnaise and too little tuna or chicken. If you love tuna, try getting just half a scoop at the cafeteria, then add some dry tuna from the salad bar. If you love chicken, opt for a grilled chicken breast. Top lunch off with a low-fat yogurt and/or glass of fat-free milk.

Keep the amount of protein to about 6 ounces for the entire day. For dinner, stick to entrées that are grilled, baked, steamed, broiled, stir-fried, or poached. Eat plenty of lean meat, such as skinless chicken or turkey breast, fish, and even on occasion a small portion of lean red meat. Choose less often foods that are fried, breaded, pan-fried, or full of cheese. For side dishes, head to the salad bar again and heap that plate with a garden patch of veggies with light dressing. As for side dishes, choose a baked potato with salsa or steamed vegetables more often than French fries, onion rings, hash browns, or fried potato skins. Avoid creamy soups and sauces that are loaded with saturated fat and calories. Take some fruit for snacking later or buy canned, single-serving fruit packed in juice for late-night snack attacks.

For breakfast, try any of these food combinations:

- Bowl of whole-grain cereal, fat-free milk, banana, and orange juice
- Toasted bagel with peanut butter
- Oatmeal with sliced peaches and grapefruit juice
- Pancakes or waffles topped with sliced strawberries and a small amount of syrup, and fat-free milk
- Hard-boiled egg, whole-wheat toast with jam, and a glass of tomato juice
- Vegetable omelet, fresh fruit salad, and fat-free milk
- Scrambled eggs and ham rolled in a flour tortilla, orange juice, and low-fat yogurt

Healthy choices for lunch include the following:

- Turkey breast or lean ham sandwich on a whole-wheat bagel with mustard and baby carrots, and low-fat yogurt topped with granola

- Baked potato topped with broccoli and salsa, an apple, and fat-free milk
- Grilled chicken sandwich on whole-wheat pita bread with honey-mustard sauce and lettuce/tomato, low-fat yogurt, and tomato juice
- Large tossed salad topped with low-fat or fat-free dressing, chickpeas, assorted fresh veggies and sunflower seeds, bread stick, and fresh strawberries
- Grilled vegetables with low-fat cheese wrapped in a flour tortilla and fresh fruit cup
- Peanut butter and jelly sandwich on whole-wheat bread, bowl of vegetable soup, and an orange
- Bean soup, pita bread, side salad, and fat-free milk

Good ideas for dinner include these:

- Grilled boneless, skinless, chicken breast topped with salsa and low-fat cheddar cheese, brown rice, green beans, and a glass of fat-free milk
- Veggie burger on a whole-grain bun, side salad, and fresh fruit
- Chicken burrito with salsa, side of vegetables, and an orange
- Broiled fish, steamed vegetables, red potatoes, and angel food cake
- Chicken fajitas with salsa and frozen yogurt
- Vegetarian chili, side salad, and fresh fruit
- Vegetable pizza, side salad, and fresh fruit
- Pasta with marinara sauce and zucchini sprinkled with parmesan cheese and fruited Jell-O

Wrong Food Choices

For many young adults, going away to college is their first experience with actually living away from home. They are now completely in charge of taking care of their own meals. There are many tempting substitutes that can take the place of good healthy meals and snacks.

Vending machines can be tempting when you are on the run from class to class. Take a look before you push the buttons. The majority of those tempting treats are full of fat and calories. For instance, a Twix bar contains 14 grams of fat and 280 calories; Peanut M&M's contain 11 grams of fat and 200 calories; a Mr. Goodbar contains 17 grams of fat and 270 calories; cheese peanut-butter crackers contain about 11 grams of fat and 210 calories; and a small bag of potato sticks contains 18 grams of fat and 250 calories. Better choices might include low-fat popcorn, pretzels, animal crackers, fig bars, low-fat granola bars, whole-wheat crackers, or low-fat breakfast bars. If you are trying to satisfy a sweet tooth, choose licorice, Lifesavers, gummy bears, or Rice Krispies Bars, and eat them in moderation. They don't contribute to your nutritional intake but they are at least generally low in fat and calories. Most of the treats found in vending machines will not hold you over for long because of their sugar content.

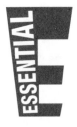

To save money and snack on something healthier than what you'll find in vending machines, carry a piece of fresh fruit or a granola bar with you for between-class snacking.

The other popular type of vending machine sells soft drinks. A regular twelve-ounce soft drink has about 150 calories, all coming from sugar. Save your money and carry a bottle of water with you. If water doesn't do it for you, choose a diet soft drink or something made with 100 percent fruit juice.

Fast-food and late-night ordering are very popular among college students. Both are quick and convenient. Remember that if you are short on cash, fast food is not exactly a bargain. Late-night munchies usually consist of ordering those extra large pizzas with everything on them or sitting down with a bag of Doritos at 2:00 A.M. Your body needs fuel throughout the day to keep your energy levels up and keep you alert. Keep in mind that calories eaten during the day are more likely to be burned off than calories eaten just before bedtime because you burn more calories when you are active. Try to stick to regular mealtimes; if you snack at night, make them light snacks. Go ahead and order pizza on occasion for a meal, but watch your toppings, which add most of the fat and calories.

Alcohol can be a culprit in those extra pounds gained as a freshman. If you are of legal drinking age, having a few occasional drinks is all right. But keep in mind that alcohol is high in calories and can also lead to late-night munchies. Another reason to drink in moderation is to avoid the effects it has on you the next day, such as headache, fatigue, nausea, and just feeling lousy. This can make it hard to concentrate in classes or complete class assignments.

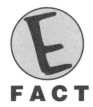

FACT

A twelve-ounce beer is 150 calories; a light beer is about 100 calories; a five-ounce serving of wine is about 105 calories; a shot (1.5 ounces) of whiskey is about 100 calories; and a 4.5 ounce Piña Colada is about 250 calories.

Healthy College Eating 101

Just because you are away from home does not mean it is time to forget all the good nutrition habits you learned as a kid. You may just need a bit of a refresher. Try these tips:

- Remember to eat three meals every day, including breakfast. It may seem like you can function on caffeine alone, but if you routinely skip meals, your brain and body will fail you when you need them most.
- Carry a water bottle with you everywhere you go. That way you can save money by not buying soda and other sweetened beverages, avoid unwanted calories, and ensure that you're well hydrated.
- Grab a piece of fruit every time you leave the dining hall, and carry it with you for a quick snack on the go.
- Take a balanced multivitamin everyday with breakfast just to ensure you are getting what you need. Don't let a supplement take the place of healthy foods, just let it round out your daily diet.
- Take a quick trip to the grocery store so you can keep quick nutritious snacks in your room: pretzels, low-fat popcorn, high-fiber crackers, low-fat breakfast bars, and unsweetened breakfast cereal. Buying snacks at the grocery store instead of the vending machine will save you money, too!
- Invest in a small dorm room refrigerator to keep other healthy snacks

such as fat-free milk, low-fat yogurt, low-fat string cheese, and fruits and vegetables. This way when you are in a pinch for time, you still have something healthy to eat.

- Avoid keeping high-calorie foods such as candy and cookies in your room. This makes it way too easy to snack on these foods all day long!

- Eat a variety of different foods. There is more than macaroni and cheese, peanut butter and jelly, and ramen noodles out there, so expand your horizons. Spend your dollar wisely, but make sure to include fruit, vegetables, whole grains, lean protein, and low-fat or fat-free dairy products every day.

- Make it your goal to try one new food each week. Experiment with vegetarian meal options such as veggie burgers. Share your meal with a friend so you can both experience something new. Or both get something different and try each other's!

Basically, take care of yourself all the way around, and get plenty of sleep and exercise. (E)

Chapter 16

Nutrition Before, During, and After Pregnancy

Nutrition should always be a priority, but when you're having a baby it becomes even more important. At this period in your life it is vital to stick to good health habits. Ensuring you receive all of the nutrients your body needs will help to promote a safe pregnancy and a healthy environment for your baby.

Pregnancy and Weight Gain

Proper weight gain is vital to a healthy baby and a safe pregnancy. A baby's birth weight is directly related to the weight you gain throughout your pregnancy. A woman who is at a healthy weight at the onset of pregnancy should expect to gain anywhere from 25 to 35 pounds during the course of the pregnancy. Women who are underweight are advised to gain 28 to 40 pounds, and women who are overweight are advised to gain 15 to 25 pounds. If you are expecting twins, your doctor may advise a weight gain of 35 to 45 pounds.

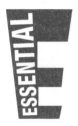

Restricting weight gain can result in a baby with a lower birth weight. Babies who are born weighing less than 5½ pounds are at greater risk for developing difficulties and illnesses than babies who weigh more.

Not only is gaining a healthy amount of weight important, but the rate at which you gain is also notable. Woman should expect about a two- to four-pound weight gain during the first trimester and about a one-pound gain per week for the remainder of the pregnancy.

Table 16-1 Where Does the Weight You Gain Go?	
Baby	7–8 pounds
Placenta	1–2 pounds
Amniotic fluid	2 pounds
Breasts	1 pound
Uterus	2 pounds
Increased blood volume	3 pounds
Body fat	5 or more pounds
Increased muscle tissue and fluid	4–7 pounds
Total	**minimum 25 pounds**

Pregnancy and Calorie Needs

Calorie needs increase during pregnancy to help support a woman's maternal body changes and the baby's proper growth and development. The RDA for energy intake during pregnancy is an additional 300 calories per day for the second and third trimester, in addition to maintenance needs. For example, if you require 2,000 calories per day to maintain your weight, you will need about 2,300 calories during pregnancy.

All the calories you consume during pregnancy should be healthy calories that contain plenty of protein, complex carbohydrates, fiber, vitamins, and minerals. Complex carbohydrates such as fruit, whole-grain starches, cereal, pasta, rice, potatoes, corn, and legumes should be the main source of energy.

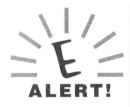

ALERT!

Dieting or skipping meals during pregnancy can have serious effects on the development of the baby. It takes more than 85,000 calories over the course of a nine-month pregnancy, in addition to the calories the mother needs for her own energy needs, to produce a healthy, well-developed baby.

Protein Power

Protein needs increase when you are pregnant to help develop the body cells of the growing baby. Other changes that are taking place in your body during pregnancy also require protein, such as the building of the placenta. You need an extra 10 grams of protein above your extra daily calories or about 70 grams of protein daily, compared with 60 grams for women who are not pregnant. Ten grams of protein is equivalent to a an ounce-and-a-half serving of lean meat, about 10 ounces of fat-free milk, or 1½ ounces of tuna canned in water.

Most women do not have a problem meeting their protein requirements. Consuming plenty of lean meats, fish, tuna, eggs, and legumes, as well as increasing your dairy servings, will ensure you meet your protein needs. If you are a vegetarian, consume a variety of legumes, grain products, eggs, low-fat or fat-free dairy products, vegetables, fruits, and soy foods to ensure proper protein intake.

Adjusting Your Eating Plan

Getting the extra calories your body needs for pregnancy just takes a small adjustment in a healthy eating plan. Adjust your eating plan using the following guidelines for the *minimum* number of servings in each food group:

- **Bread, cereal, rice, and pasta group:** 6–7 (or more) servings daily
- **Vegetable and fruit groups:** 5 or more servings daily
- **Milk, yogurt, and cheese group:** 2–3 servings daily
- **Meat, poultry, fish, dried beans, eggs, and nut group:** 5–7 ounces daily
- **Unsaturated fats:** 3 servings daily

Also be aware of increased fluid needs. Water is an important nutrient and is essential for the nourishment that passes through the placenta to the baby. Drink at least 8 to 12 cups daily and more if you are thirsty.

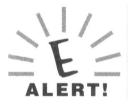

Raw foods can increase your risk for bacterial infection. Avoid anything raw, including sushi and other raw seafood, undercooked meat or poultry, beef tartar, raw or unpasteurized milk, soft-cooked or poached eggs, and raw eggs (possibly found in eggnog).

Vitamin and Mineral Needs

Vitamin and mineral needs also increase with pregnancy. Unlike calorie needs, your increased need for vitamins and minerals is immediate. Certain ones are especially important such as folate, calcium, and iron.

Folate

Folate is especially important for women during the first three months of pregnancy. The body uses folate to manufacture new cells and genetic material. During pregnancy, folate helps develop the neural tube, which becomes the baby's spine. Because most women do not know that they are pregnant immediately, and because the neural tube and brain begin to form so soon after conception, taking enough folate on a regular basis is important if you are of childbearing age. Taking enough folate can help to greatly reduce the risk of neural tube birth defects like spina bifida and birth defects of the brain (anencephaly). The National Academy of Sciences recommends women of childbearing age get 400 micrograms (mcg) of folate each day especially one month prior to conception.

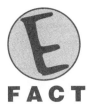

FACT

National surveys show that the average folic acid intake by women of childbearing age is about 230 micrograms daily. Folic acid intake should be kept below 1,000 micrograms per day to avoid excessive intake.

Most women get folic acid daily through fortified products and other foods. To get more folic acid in their diets, women anticipating pregnancy should eat more citrus fruits and juices, leafy dark-green vegetables, legumes, and fortified breakfast cereals. To ensure adequate intake, woman can take a multivitamin that contains folic acid in addition to a healthy diet.

Not all vitamin supplements contain folic acid, so check the label to make sure about the amount. Also, not all multivitamin supplements are optimal before or during pregnancy. Pregnant women and those anticipating pregnancy should consult their doctor for advice about taking folic acid or any other vitamin or mineral supplement.

Vitamin A

Vitamin A is important for promoting growth and health of cells and tissues throughout your body and the baby's. A healthy diet should provide enough vitamin A during pregnancy so there is no need for a supplement.

New research has shown that consuming too much vitamin A, in excess of 10,000 IU daily, may increase the risk of birth defects. This is twice the RDA. Eating foods such as fruits and vegetables that are high in beta-carotene is not a problem because beta-carotene does not convert to vitamin A when blood levels of vitamin A are at normal levels.

Other Vitamins

With your increase in calorie intake, your increased need for most of the B vitamins will be met through your dietary intake. Vitamin B_{12} is found in animal foods such as milk, eggs, meat, and cheese. Women who are vegetarian and don't consume any type of animal foods need to make sure they consume a reliable source of vitamin B_{12}, such as fortified breakfast cereals and/or a B_{12} supplement. If you don't feel you are meeting your B_{12} needs, talk to your doctor before taking supplements.

Vitamin C needs increase slightly but can be met easily with a glass of orange juice, an orange, or another citrus fruit. Vitamin C is important because it helps the body absorb iron from plant sources, and iron needs almost double during pregnancy.

Vitamin D is essential because it helps the body to absorb extra needed calcium. A glass of vitamin-D fortified milk will take care of your extra needs. For vegetarians who do not consume dairy products, your doctor may prescribe a supplement. Make sure your doctor knows your eating habits!

Pumping Up Calcium and Iron

Two minerals that deserve special attention are calcium and iron. If you don't consume enough of either of these minerals through your pregnancy, the baby will actually use the calcium in your bones and the iron in your blood.

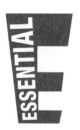

The estimated calcium needs for pregnant girls under eighteen is 1,300 mg per day. For pregnant adult women aged nineteen to fifty, the recommended intake is 1,000 mg per day. There is also an Upper Tolerable Limit for pregnant women set at 2,500 mg per day.

Although it is important to get calcium throughout your life, it is especially important during pregnancy. Calcium helps ensure that your bone mass is preserved while the baby's skeleton develops normally.

Consuming plenty of calcium before, during, and after pregnancy can also help reduce your risk for osteoporosis later in life. Good sources of calcium include dairy products and some green leafy vegetables. If you are vegetarian or lactose intolerant and do not consume dairy products, consume plenty of other good calcium sources, such as calcium-fortified orange juice or calcium-fortified soy milk, along with special lactose-reduced products.

An increase in the blood volume of a pregnant woman greatly increases her iron needs. A woman's need for iron increases to 30 mg per day. Several foods supply iron, including meat, poultry, fish, legumes, and whole-grain and enriched grain products. Iron needs during pregnancy can be more difficult to meet because iron isn't always absorbed well, and many women have low iron stores before they get pregnant. Most prenatal vitamins contain iron, and your doctor may also prescribe an iron supplement. Keep in mind, though, that supplements are just to help out; you still need to eat a diet rich in iron. Iron from plant sources is not as easily absorbed as that from animal sources. Eating a good source of vitamin C, such as citrus fruits or juices, broccoli, tomatoes, or kiwi with meals will help the body absorb the iron in the foods that you eat. The absorption of iron from supplements is best when the stomach is empty or when taken with juice containing vitamin C.

Handling the Discomforts of Pregnancy

Because of the many changes that are going on in your body during pregnancy, you may feel the occasional discomfort of morning sickness, constipation, heartburn, and swelling.

The first discomfort most pregnant women experience is morning sickness. For many women this is not just something that takes place in the morning. Many women feel sick all day long.

There is no exact known reason why some women get morning sickness so much worse than others or why women get morning sickness at all. For some women, but not all, the feeling of nausea will gradually begin to improve at around twelve to fourteen weeks of pregnancy.

If you know for sure that your nausea is normal morning sickness, you can follow some of these tips to help ease your discomfort:

- Eat small, frequent meals, every two hours (even through the night, if you can).
- Eat a snack before going to bed at night such as cheese and crackers, peanut butter on bread, or cereal and milk.
- Eat starchy foods such as dry crackers, graham crackers, dry cereal, or plain toast before getting out of bed in the morning, and get out of bed slowly.
- Eat a high-carbohydrate diet with foods such as dry toast, fruit, bagels, baked potato, pasta, whole-grain breakfast cereals, rice, vegetables, and other easy-to-digest carbohydrates. Nibble on small amounts of these foods throughout the day.
- Avoid strong smells, strong food flavors, and spicy foods. Pregnant women often have an exaggerated sense of smell, making strong odors unappealing.
- Some women find cold foods easier to tolerate than hot foods.
- Avoid high-fat and fried foods. They can sit in your stomach longer, making your nausea worse.
- Nausea is worsened by fatigue, so make sure you're getting enough rest at night, and try to take naps during the day.
- If you are taking any type of vitamin or mineral supplement, take them with meals or snacks. If you are taking iron pills, try taking them with a light snack or two hours after a meal with some ginger ale or juice.
- Listen to your body, and let taste and tolerance be your guide.

ALERT!

If you begin to experience episodes of vomiting more than twice daily, contact your doctor immediately.

Constipation can be another discomfort that is very normal during pregnancy. Hormonal changes relax muscles to accommodate the expanded uterus and this can cause a slowdown in the action of your intestine. This as well as iron supplements can be the culprits of aggravating constipation. To help ease this discomfort, try the following:

- Drink plenty of fluids. In addition to water, include other fluids like milk and juice.
- Eat a diet rich in fiber. Consume at least five servings of fruits and vegetables daily; eat whole-grain breads, cereals, rice, and pasta; and try including legumes or dry beans at least a few times a week.
- Try foods that have natural laxative effects, such as dried prunes, prune juice, and figs.
- Be as physically active as possible with activities such as walking and swimming. Regular activity can help stimulate normal bowel function. Talk to your doctor about safe activities and exercise.

Heartburn and acid reflux can be other nagging discomforts of pregnancy, especially during the last three months. Heartburn usually occurs because the baby is putting pressure on the digestive organs. Acid reflux happens because the valve between your stomach and esophagus becomes more relaxed, making it easier for food to occasionally reverse direction.

To help relieve these discomforts, try these tips:

- Eat small, frequent meals, every few hours.
- Relax and eat your food slowly.
- Go easy on spicy or highly seasoned foods, as well as rich, fried, or fatty foods.
- Limit fluids with your meals, but increase your fluids between meals.
- Cut down on caffeine. For some women, caffeine can cause nausea and heartburn.
- After eating, walk or stay seated to help gastric juices to flow in the right direction.
- Sleep with your head elevated.
- Wear clothes that are loose and comfortable, as opposed to tight and restricting.

- Keep a log of the foods you eat to help you track certain foods that may be triggering your heartburn.
- Do not take antacids without consulting your doctor first.

Swelling can also cause some discomfort during pregnancy, especially during the last three months. Your body retains water primarily in your feet, ankles, and hands as a reservoir for the expanded blood volume.

To help relieve some of the discomforts of water retention, try these tips:

- Lie down and elevate your feet on a pillow.
- Wear comfortable shoes, and try not to stand for long periods.
- Avoid tight-fitting clothes.
- Do not limit your fluid intake; continue to drink plenty of fluids, including water.
- There is rarely a need to reduce your sodium intake unless you are consuming much more than the recommended levels of 2,400 mg per day.

If your swelling is excessive, it could be a sign of complications like eclampsia or toxemia. With these conditions you may have other symptoms such as high blood pressure, sudden weight gain, headaches, and abdominal pain. Consult your doctor immediately if you have any of these symptoms.

Pregnancy and Diabetes

Gestational diabetes occurs in approximately 4 percent of all pregnancies. Gestational diabetes is distinguished by an elevated glucose, or blood sugar level, during pregnancy. Women are routinely tested between the twenty-fourth and twenty-eighth weeks of pregnancy to make sure they are not showing symptoms of gestational diabetes. The risk is usually higher for women who have a family history of diabetes, who are overweight, and who have had problem pregnancies in the past. Gestational diabetes is usually diagnosed during the second or third trimester of pregnancy. Women who have known diabetes before pregnancy are not diagnosed as having gestational diabetes. This type of diabetes disappears in 90 percent of women after giving birth.

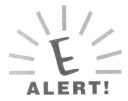

ALERT!

Women who experience gestational diabetes are at an increased risk, as much as 60 percent, for developing Type 2 diabetes later. Women can decrease their risk by maintaining a healthy weight after their pregnancy.

The nutritional goals for women with gestational diabetes are to provide adequate calories, optimal nutrition, and normalized blood sugar levels. Monitoring blood sugar on a regular basis is essential to knowing if normal blood sugar levels are being achieved. Guidelines for treating this type of diabetes varies and is very individualized, but one constant recommendation is limiting carbohydrate intake at breakfast. Most women with gestational diabetes cannot tolerate large amounts of carbohydrates in the morning but are generally able to tolerate them later in the day. Foods high in total amounts of carbohydrate are also limited. Eating small, frequent meals throughout the day as well as getting regular exercise can also help to normalize blood sugar levels during pregnancy.

If you are diagnosed with gestational diabetes, your doctor and/or a dietitian should work with you closely to help you develop a meal and lifestyle plan that will help you to control your blood sugar levels.

For Women Who Breastfeed

If you are breastfeeding, good nutrition after giving birth is just as important as it was before. The fuel supply that helps produce your breast milk comes from energy stored as body fat during your pregnancy and from extra energy from food choices. Your body uses about 100 to 150 additional calories per day to produce breast milk. While breastfeeding, a woman needs an additional 500 calories per day, beyond nonpregnancy maintenance needs. In other words, if you needed 2,000 calories to maintain your weight before pregnancy, you need 2,700 calories per day while you are breastfeeding. Trying to lose weight through a strict weight-loss regimen is not recommended while you are breastfeeding. If your caloric intake goes lower than 1,800 calories, you probably will not get enough of all the nutrients your body needs for proper breastfeeding.

As in pregnancy, the need for most nutrients increases while breastfeeding. It is important to pay extra close attention to your protein, calcium, magnesium, zinc, vitamin B_{12}, vitamin D, folate, and vitamin B_6 intake. If your nutrient intake is low, you can still produce breast milk sufficient enough to support your baby's health but only at the expense of your own body's nutrient reserves. Also remember your fluid intake during this time. Continue to get at least 8 to 12 cups of fluids daily and more if you are thirsty.

Alcohol can pass into breast milk so it is not advised during breastfeeding. It is also advised that you not smoke. Nicotine does pass into breast milk. It can reduce your milk supply and increase your baby's risk for developing colic or a sinus infection. If you do smoke, avoid smoking for two and a half hours before nursing, and never smoke around the baby. Some medications, both prescription and over-the-counter, can be passed through breast milk. It is advised to consult your physician before taking any type of medication when breastfeeding.

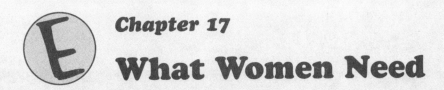

Chapter 17

What Women Need

The nutritional needs of women change over their life spans. In contrast, men's nutritional needs do not change much. The American Dietetic Association states, "Nutrition is involved in the etiology or treatment of half of the 10 leading causes of death in women."

Nutrition and Menstruation

The menstrual cycle in a woman is a delicate interaction of hormones and physiological responses. The menstrual cycle is the body's way of preparing itself every month for a possible pregnancy. As women of childbearing age go through menstruation, overall nutrition is an important issue.

Boosting Iron

During a woman's years of menstruation, iron needs are a special nutritional concern. On average, women lose about ¼ cup of blood at each menstrual cycle; women with a heavier flow may even lose more. Since iron travels through the blood, some of it is lost with the loss of blood.

Women of childbearing age have an RDA of 15 mg per day for iron, which doubles with pregnancy. Women over fifty-one have a lower RDA of 10 mg per day because most of them have reached menopause and are no longer losing blood (and therefore iron) each month.

It is common for women of childbearing age to become iron deficient. A deficiency of iron can cause symptoms that include fatigue and weakness. Deficiency can also lead to anemia. The combination of iron lost through the menstrual cycle, a low dietary intake of iron, frequent dieting, and a low intake of vitamin C all contribute to the problem of iron deficiency.

It is helpful not only to eat iron-rich foods but also to take a multivitamin supplement that contains iron. Many supplements contain iron and are designed for women with that in mind. However, it is a good idea to check your supplement to make sure it contains iron.

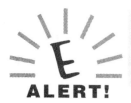

ALERT!

If you take both an iron and calcium supplement, take them separately, at different times of the day. They will both be better absorbed if taken on their own.

Iron can be found in both animal products and plant sources, but the iron from meat is better absorbed than that in plant foods. Certain nutrients, such as vitamin C, can help enhance the absorption of iron from plant sources. So you can increase the amount of iron the body can use from iron-containing plant foods by, for example, drinking a glass of orange juice. Good sources of iron include meat, poultry, fish, fortified cereal, enriched rice, and legumes.

Premenstrual Syndrome (PMS)

Premenstrual Syndrome, or PMS, is a condition that afflicts many women. This condition can have several symptoms and varying degrees of severity from woman to woman. The exact cause of PMS is not completely understood, though experts do believe that hormones such as progesterone, estrogen, and testosterone are probably involved. A change in the level of serotonin in the brain is also believed to be related to the occurrence of PMS. For most women the symptoms of PMS seem to appear after ovulation, or about fourteen days into the cycle, and disappear two weeks later, as the menstrual period starts. PMS is closely tied with mood swings, bloating from water retention, tender breasts, headaches, temporary weight gain, and food cravings.

Avoiding certain foods can help. Some of the following foods may exacerbate your symptoms: caffeine, simple sugars, salt or sodium, fats, and alcohol.

Even though food cravings and other symptoms may be a predictable part of PMS, some things can be done to help relieve some symptoms. Foods that may help to relieve some symptoms include complex carbohydrates and high-calcium foods. Stick to a diet that includes plenty of fresh fruits and vegetables, whole-grain products, non-fat dairy products, lean fish, and poultry; also drink plenty of water. Besides a healthy diet, be sure to exercise regularly. Exercise can help release tension and anxiety, and it promotes the release of endorphins, which naturally sedate you.

There are many supplements as well as claims about certain vitamins that supposedly help to relieve the effects of PMS. At one time vitamin B_6 was believed to help relieve PMS symptoms, but solid evidence was never found, and taking too much B_6 was harming many women. To get the possible benefits of B_6, consume foods rich in the vitamin, including fish, chicken, soy foods, broccoli, bananas, cantaloupe, and spinach. Until more is known, your best bet in helping relieve PMS symptoms is to follow some general guidelines. Eat an overall healthy diet, lead an active lifestyle, get plenty of sleep, and consult your doctor if needed.

Nutrition and Menopause

Menopause is the natural part of a women's lifecycle when the menstrual period stops. It is sometimes called "the change of life" and is a unique and personal experience for every woman.

Menopause is a natural life event that marks the end of the child-bearing years for women. In technical terms, menopause occurs when the ovaries run out of eggs and decrease the production of the sex hormone estrogen, progesterone, and androgen. Women experience menopause at various ages, but most go through it around age fifty. It is considered an early menopause at any age younger than forty to forty-five.

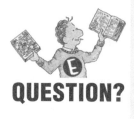

QUESTION?

Are there other factors that will effect the age at which I hit menopause?
Genetics is definitely a key factor, so knowing your family history may give you a clue. Also, cigarette smoking can cause menopause to occur two years earlier for women who smoke than for nonsmoking women.

Changes and signs of menopause include the following:

- Hot flashes (sudden warm feeling, sometimes with blushing)
- Night sweats (hot flashes that occur usually at night and can often disrupt sleep)
- Fatigue (probably from disrupted sleep patterns)
- Mood swings
- Early-morning awakening
- Vaginal dryness

- Fluctuations in sexual desire or response
- Difficulty sleeping

Many of the symptoms as well as health problems of menopause are due to the decreasing levels of estrogen. Treatment with estrogen (estrogen replacement therapy, or ERT) or with estrogen and progestin (hormone replacement therapy, HRT) has been used to help relieve some of these symptoms and supposedly decrease the risk for certain health problems such as heart disease and stroke. Approximately 25 percent or 8 million American menopausal women currently take ERT or HRT. Taking ERT or HRT may help to reduce symptoms of menopause but it is now uncertain whether the risks outweigh the benefits. There is doubt as to whether they really do decrease the risks of certain health problems and there are contraindications in taking HRT for women who have a history of cancer. Taking HRT and ERT is an extremely complicated issue with many pros and cons. Every woman should assess her own personal needs and discuss her options with her doctor. If you're taking these replacements, it is important to have regular medical check-ups.

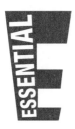

An ongoing study being done by the National Institutes of Health called the Women's Health Initiative (WHI) is studying the effects of both ERT and HRT on women. Due to their recent findings, they have asked the women in the study to stop using HRT. They concluded that HRT does not prevent heart disease and is not beneficial overall. The jury is still out on the benefits of taking estrogen (ERT) alone. The scientists at WHI are continuing to study and analyze the use of ERT and HRT. You can find updated information at ✑*http://www.nih.gov* and ✑*http://www.whi.org.*

Current research is now examining soy foods as an alternative treatment for the symptoms of menopause. These soy foods contain phytoestrogen (also called isoflavones), a plant hormone similar to estrogen. Research is still in its beginning stages, and much more needs to be established before any conclusions can be made.

Health Issues and Menopause

At least two major health problems can develop in women in the years after menopause: heart disease and osteoporosis. A decrease in hormone production is most likely the cause of these conditions at that stage in life. The years following menopause can be healthy years, depending on how you take care of yourself. Not all women will develop heart disease or osteoporosis after menopause. Many lifestyle factors can affect your heart and your bones that have nothing to do with estrogen levels. The key to helping prevent heart disease and osteoporosis is lifestyle change, with nutrition and physical activity as major components.

Weight Gain in Menopause

Perimenopause, which leads to menopause, marks the beginning of the end of the menstrual cycle. In this stage, which spans from five to ten years, estrogen levels begin to decline, ovulation becomes less regular and weight gain tends to become a problem. Some women who have struggled with just a few extra pounds often find themselves struggling harder against weight gain during perimenopause. Even women who have generally stayed in a healthy weight range for many years suddenly find themselves having to work a lot harder to stay there. Some experts believe that the reason for the weight problems is the fluctuation in hormone levels, while others suggest it is an age-related decline in muscle mass that ultimately decreases metabolism. As with weight loss at any stage of life, dieting isn't the only answer. The key is lifestyle change and exercise combined. Experts feel that if you have not been exercising throughout life, perimenopause is the time when you should really begin. At this point in your life you need to develop more muscle mass through exercise to achieve a higher, fat-burning metabolic rate that can help you lose extra pounds and help you to stay at a healthy weight.

Women and Heart Disease

There are many serious types of health concerns that affect women. None is more serious than heart disease, the nation's leading killer. The

American Heart Association says that "nearly one million people die from heart disease yearly." Heart disease is often thought of as a man's disease, but that is a misconception. Even though breast cancer is most often quoted as the number one cause of death in women, nearly six times as many women die from heart disease. In 1996, women's deaths from heart disease outpaced men's by 505,930 to 453,297. The facts tell it all: one in nine women over age forty-five and one in three women over sixty-five have coronary heart disease. Approximately half of all women will eventually develop some form of heart disease.

Up until menopause, estrogen reduces the likelihood of plaque buildup in the arteries and acts as protection from heart disease.

After menopause, a woman's risk steadily increases for developing coronary artery disease, or CAD, a condition where the veins and arteries leading to the heart become narrowed and/or blocked by plaque. Heart attack and stroke are caused by CAD, in most cases.

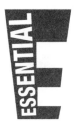

Estrogen helps to raise HDL cholesterol (good cholesterol), which helps remove LDL cholesterol (the bad cholesterol) that contributes to the accumulation of fat deposits called plaque along artery walls.

Women need to concentrate on making heart-healthy choices throughout life but especially in the years after menopause. It is important to eat a diet that is low in total fat, saturated fat, and cholesterol; eat plenty of grain products, vegetables, and fruits; stay physically active; keep a healthy weight; control stress levels; go easy on sodium; and consult with a doctor about hormone replacement therapy.

Osteoporosis

Osteoporosis afflicts more than 8 million women and 2 million men. More than 80 percent of osteoporosis sufferers are women; osteoporosis affects half of all women over the age of fifty and almost 90 percent of those over the age of seventy-five. Five to 20 percent of women die each year due to osteoporosis-related complications. Osteoporosis is a brittle-bone disease that increases the risk of bone fractures later in life.

Your Risks for Osteoporosis

Menopause is the single greatest risk for osteoporosis; others include gender, age, family history, hormone deficiencies, low calcium intake, excessive alcohol and caffeine consumption, and cigarette smoking. Estrogen helps prevent bone loss and works together with calcium and other hormones and minerals to help build bones. When women hit menopause and are not making as much estrogen, their risk for osteoporosis increases. The key is trying to prevent osteoporosis in your younger years instead of treating it after menopause. The stronger and healthier your bones are when you enter menopause, the more bone mass you will have to sustain you as you age.

Bone loss varies from woman to woman. Osteoporosis prevention should include a balanced diet rich in calcium and vitamin D. From childhood through early adulthood, adequate calcium helps build bone mass; in the late postmenopausal years, eating plenty of calcium-rich foods and taking a calcium supplement can help slow bone loss. Experts also recommend participating in weight-bearing type exercises, such as walking and avoiding smoking and excessive caffeine intake.

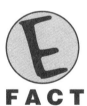

FACT

The RDA for women after menopause, not taking hormone replacement therapy, is 1,500 mg of calcium daily; for women who do take HRT, the RDA is 1,200 mg of calcium.

How to Handle Osteoporosis

Osteoporosis has no actual cure, but you can take some treatments and preventive measures to help slow or reverse bone loss and help prevent fractures. Try some of these tips:

- Increase your calcium intake to 1,000–1,500 mg per day. As you age, your body absorbs and uses calcium less efficiently. Foods high in calcium include dairy foods, green leafy vegetables, shellfish, sardines with bones, oysters, brazil nuts, fortified tofu, and almonds. Many foods are available on the market today that are fortified with calcium, such as orange juice, breads, breakfast cereals, and soy milk.

- Weight-bearing exercise that actually puts weight on your bones—such as weight resistance training, walking, jogging, aerobic dance, or tennis—can help promote bone health.
- Consult your doctor about whether taking hormone replacement therapy (HRT) is right for you. Combined with exercise and adequate calcium, HRT may help prevent bone loss, but the benefits may not outweight the risks.
- Reduce your caffeine intake (about 40 mg extra dietary calcium is needed to offset the amount of calcium lost from one cup of coffee).
- Drink alcohol in moderation. People who drink heavily have less bone mass and lose bone more rapidly.
- Stop smoking. People who smoke have a greater risk of fracture. Also, women who smoke have lower estrogen levels, which is what helps protect you from osteoporosis.

It is advised that women be evaluated for osteoporosis if they fracture easily, are sixty-five or older, or are menopausal with other risk factors. If left completely untreated, a postmenopausal woman can lose 10 to 40 percent of bone mass between the ages of fifty and sixty.

Breast Cancer

Cancer is the second leading cause of death in American women. According to the National Cancer Institute, "Other than skin cancer, breast cancer is the most common type of cancer among women in the United States. More than 180,000 women are diagnosed with breast cancer each year." The exact cause of breast cancer as well as many other types of cancers is not yet known. However, studies do show that the risk of breast cancer increases greatly in older women and seems more uncommon in women under the age of thirty-five. In fact, most cases of breast cancer occur in women over fifty, and the risk is even higher in women over sixty. Also, breast cancer occurs more often in white women than African-American or Asian women.

Diet and Breast Cancer

Lifestyle factors play a potential role in the etiology of breast cancer. More specifically, it's the amount and type of fat consumed; the carotenoid, phytochemical, and flavonoid content of the diet; and lifestyle conditions, such as consuming too many calories and physical inactivity, that may affect the risk of contracting breast cancer. A plant-based diet adequate in vegetables, fruits, and phytochemicals is to some degree protective against breast cancer. Carotenoids and flavonoids, which are substances found in vegetables and fruits, may have a protective effect against cancers such as breast cancer. Soy foods have also received recent attention due to their probable cancer-fighting properties. The isoflavone genistein, a phytoestrogen found in soy foods, is believed to possess some anticancer properties. In addition to providing protective substances, plant-based diets provide more fiber, which may offer protection against breast cancer. As with any type of cancer, a healthy diet and healthy lifestyle are important steps in taking preventive measures.

Risk Factors for Breast Cancer

Several factors can increase your risk for getting breast cancer:

- A history of breast cancer increases your risk of getting it in the other breast.
- Having a family history of breast cancer.
- Evidence suggests that the longer a woman is exposed to estrogen (estrogen made by the body, taken as a drug, or delivered by a patch), the higher risk they run for breast cancer. The risk is somewhat increased among women who began menstruating at an earlier age (before age twelve), experienced menopause late (after age fifty-five), never had children, or took HRT for long periods of time. Each of these factors increases the amount of time a woman's body is exposed to estrogen.
- Women who have their first child late (after about age thirty) have a greater chance of developing breast cancer than women who have a child at a younger age.

- Having breast radiation therapy before age thirty.
- Being overweight or obese.
- Poor dietary intake.
- Studies suggest a slightly higher risk among women who drink alcohol.

Regular screenings for breast cancer have been shown to help decrease the number of deaths from breast cancer. Women should take an active part in early detection by scheduling regular mammograms and clinical breast exams as well as performing breast self-exams.

Obesity and Overweight in Women

Women seem to be especially vulnerable to weight gain during three key periods of their lives: at the beginning of their menstrual cycle, after pregnancy, and after menopause. Women who are obese (with a BMI greater than 30) or overweight (BMI of 25–29.9) are at greater risk for gallbladder disease, respiratory disease, gout, sleep apnea, osteoarthritis, and several types of cancer. Overweight and obesity are also linked to a higher risk of hypertension, high cholesterol, and Type 2 diabetes, which all contribute to mortality in women. Furthermore, being obese or overweight is associated with poor pregnancy outcome, miscarriage, infertility, and polycystic ovarian syndrome.

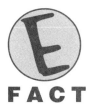

FACT

According to the U.S. Surgeon General, overweight and obesity are increasing in both men and women. The latest estimates are that 34 percent of U.S. adults aged twenty to seventy-four are overweight, and an additional 27 percent are obese. About half of all women aged twenty to seventy-four are overweight or obese. The percentages of obese women among African-, Native-, and Mexican-American women are even higher.

Besides increasing the risk for several health problems, overweight and obesity place a great psychological burden on women. People who are obese can suffer from prejudice in society and enjoy a reduced quality of life. Eating disorders and perceptions of altered body images can begin early in a woman's life and continue throughout most of her life. Many women end up being dissatisfied with their bodies, having low self-esteem, and engaging in phases of dieting throughout life. Leading a healthy lifestyle that includes a healthy diet and plenty of physical activity is essential for women to reach and maintain a healthy weight.

Eating Disorders

Eating disorders are complex and chronic illnesses that tend to be misdiagnosed and highly misunderstood. Some of the most common eating disorders include anorexia nervosa, bulimia nervosa, and binge eating. Another type of disorder under examination is extreme exercise to control weight. All of these disorders are on the rise in the United States and worldwide.

Many factors play a role in the development of an eating disorder, including personality, self-esteem, genetics, environment, and body chemistry.

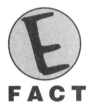

FACT

Women seem to make up more than 90 percent of the people who have eating disorders. It is estimated that in the United States, at least 5 to 10 million females and 1 million males between the ages of fourteen and twenty-five have an eating disorder.

Eating disorders should be taken seriously. They require the help of a health-care provider as soon as symptoms begin to surface.

Anorexia Nervosa

Anorexia nervosa is an eating disorder characterized by a person who literally starves himself or herself by eating little to no food. People who have this condition have a strong fear of body fat and weight gain. Anorexics refuse to eat. They exhibit an intense desire to be unrealistically thin, consistently repeat attempts at dieting, and experience excessive weight loss. To maintain their abnormally low body weight, anorexics may diet, fast, or overexercise. People with anorexia will do just about anything to get or stay thin, such as self-induced vomiting and/or the misuse of laxative, diuretics, or enemas. People with anorexia see themselves as fat even though they are extremely thin.

One of the most dangerous hazards of anorexia is starvation. The body reacts to starvation by extreme thinness, brittle nails and hair, dry skin, a slow pulse, cold intolerance, constipation, and occasional diarrhea. In addition, a person may experience mild anemia, a loss of muscle mass, loss of the menstrual cycle, and swelling of joints. Malnutrition caused by anorexia may result in irregular heart rhythms and heart failure. The lack of nutrients can place anorexics at even more health risks such as the lack of calcium, which places them at increased risk for osteoporosis both during their illness and in later life. Many anorexics suffer with clinical depression, anxiety, personality disorders, and/or substance abuse. Unfortunately, many more are also at risk for suicide. It is estimated that one in ten anorexics will die from starvation, heart attack, or other serious medical complication, making this disorder's death rate among the highest for a psychiatric disease.

A person with anorexia may do the following:

- Eat only certain or "safe" foods, usually those with very few calories and/or little fat.
- Adopt strange rituals when eating, such as cutting food into very small pieces.
- Spend more time playing or pushing food around on the plate than actually eating it.
- Cook meals for others without eating any.
- Engage in exercise compulsively.
- Dress in layers to hide excessive weight loss.
- Become more isolated, spending less time with family and friends.

Bulimia Nervosa

Bulimia nervosa is an eating disorder characterized by a person who binges, or consumes a very large amount of food all at once and then purges. Purging means forcing yourself to vomit, take laxatives, or diuretics (water pills). Bulimics may also fast or use excessive exercise as a means of ridding the body of what they ate during a binge. Their binge eating is usually very secretive and uncontrolled. As with anorexia nervosa, those with bulimia are overly concerned with food, body weight, and shape.

Binge sessions can occur one or twice a week to several times per day and can be triggered by a wide range of emotions. With bulimia, the disorder can be constant or have periods of remission.

Medical complications that are attributed to bulimia nervosa usually result from an imbalance of electrolytes from repeated vomiting. There is usually a loss of potassium, which can damage the heart muscle, and an increased risk of heart attack. Repeated vomiting can also cause an inflammation of the esophagus and erosion of tooth enamel as well as damage to salivary glands.

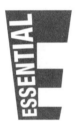

Bulimia is different from anorexia in that many individuals with bulimia "binge and purge" in secret and maintain normal or above normal body weight, so they can often hide the disorder from others for years.

Like those with anorexia, many people with bulimia suffer from clinical depression and anxiety as well as obsessive-compulsive disorder and other mental illnesses.

A person with bulimia may do the following:

- Become very secretive about food, usually planning the next binge session.
- Take frequent trips to the bathroom, especially right after eating.
- Steal food and/or hide it in strange places.
- Engage in compulsive exercising.

Binge Eating Disorder

Binge eating disorder is probably one of the most common types of eating disorders and is more common in women than in men. A majority of the people who are afflicted with this disorder are overweight or obese, but not all. A binge eating disorder results in a person's inability to control the desire to overeat. Most people with this disorder keep it an exclusive secret. Unlike bulimia, people with a binge eating disorder do not purge their food. Binge eating does show up in bulimia.

People with binge eating disorder do not eat highly nutritious diets and are at a greater risk for illness because they may not be getting the correct nutrients. They usually eat large amounts of fats and sugars, which don't have a lot of vitamins or minerals.

People with binge eating disorder may do the following:

- Feel their eating is out of control.
- Eat what most people would think is an unusually large amount of food.
- Eat much more quickly than usual during binge episodes.
- Eat until so full they are uncomfortable.
- Eat large amounts of food, even when they are not really hungry.
- Eat alone because they are embarrassed about the amount they eat.
- Feel disgusted, depressed, or guilty after overeating.

People with binge eating disorder should be advised to get immediate help from a mental health professional. For help with weight loss, they should also be advised to seek out help from a registered dietitian. Even those who are not overweight are usually upset by their binge eating, so treatment can help them.

Treating Eating Disorders

There are several different ways to treat eating disorders and presently there is no universally accepted standard of treatment. It is ideal to have an integrated approach to treatment, including the skills of registered dietitians, mental health professionals, endocrinologists, and other medical doctors. Types of psychotherapy that are often used include cognitive-behavioral therapy, interpersonal psychotherapy, and family and group therapy. Drug therapy, such as antidepressants, may be helpful for some people.

If an individual displays any of the characteristics described here for any type of eating disorder, he or she should be taken to a physician, nutritionist, or other professional with expertise in diagnosing eating disorders as soon as possible.

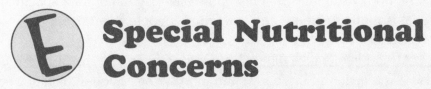

Chapter 18

Special Nutritional Concerns

Eating can be a particular challenge for those with special health concerns. Living a healthy lifestyle is the best approach to promoting health and possibly slowing or preventing the course of several health problems. Learning how to comfortably and confidently live with a special health or nutritional concern can make a huge difference in the quality of one's life.

Understanding Food Allergies

About one in three adults consider themselves to have a milk allergy. However the reality is that less than 2 percent of all adults have an actual food allergy of *any* kind. Food allergies are frequently misconceived as a reaction or intolerance to a certain food. A true food allergy is the result of the body's immune system abnormally responding to a specific food. What is more common, and what more people suffer from, are food intolerances.

A food intolerance differs from a food allergy in that it does not cause a reaction in the body's immune system. Food intolerances can result from failure of the body to digest the consumed food properly. Most people with intolerances can eat small amounts of the food without problems.

When a true food allergy occurs, proteins from a specific food—called antigens or allergens—set off a chain of immune system reactions. When a person eats a food he or she is allergic to, the body makes antibodies to protect itself. These antibodies trigger the release of body chemicals such as histamines, which cause uncomfortable allergic symptoms. The confusion arises between allergies and intolerances because symptoms of both can resemble each other. The best way to determine an allergy from an intolerance is not to self-diagnose but to be actually tested and diagnosed by a board-certified allergist. If you do have a true food allergy, is important to know for sure that you are able to stay away from the offending foods. Unlike food intolerances, food allergies can be tested for because they cause changes in the immune system. People with a family history of allergies are at higher risk of developing one. Most food allergies surface in early childhood, and most are outgrown as the child gets older.

Symptoms

Food allergies can trigger different physical responses that vary individually. Some of the symptoms can be due to other causes; therefore, medical evaluation is essential. The histamines that are responsible for the multiple symptoms of an allergic reaction can range from minor sneezes and sniffles to anaphylaxis, a life-threatening reaction.

Reactions from foods can occur within second or hours after eating a food. Common food allergy symptoms can include the following:

- Swelling of lips, mouth, tongue, face, and/or throat
- Hives and/or rash
- Sneezing and/or nasal congestion
- Chronic coughing
- Asthma

- Nausea
- Abdominal pain and bloating
- Vomiting
- Diarrhea
- Cramping
- Gas

Any food can cause a reaction, but foods that are more likely to cause physical reactions include milk, nuts, eggs, soy, peas, fish, and shellfish. Food allergies from soy, milk, wheat, and eggs are usually outgrown. Food allergies from peanuts, nuts, fish, and shellfish are less frequently outgrown.

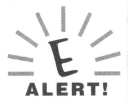
ALERT!

If you or a family member has experienced severe food reactions in the past, it is vital to plan in advance how you might handle an accidental ingestion of the trigger food. You should wear an identification necklace or bracelet to alert others to your severe allergy, and you should carry epinephrine (adrenaline) to be quickly injected to help counter the allergen.

For the majority of people with food allergies, the symptoms are just more uncomfortable than dangerous. In some rare cases, though, reactions are much more life threatening. Some experience an anaphylactic reaction, which often happens within a few seconds or minutes after eating the food. The symptoms may include any combination of skin reactions; nose, throat, and lung reactions; and stomach and intestinal reactions. Symptoms can include nausea, diarrhea, chest pain, extreme itching, sweating, asthma, rapid or irregular heart beat, low blood pressure, and shock. Immediate medical attention is essential, and without it death can occur. Foods that are most likely to cause anaphylactic reactions include peanuts and tree nuts, eggs, and shellfish.

Diagnosing

If you have symptoms or suspect any type of food allergy, a board-certified allergist should diagnose you properly. A diagnosis can include a medical history, a physical exam, keeping a food diary, an elimination diet, and/or laboratory testing.

Keeping a food diary and tracking any symptoms experienced for two to four weeks is one technique. This can be helpful in pinpointing which foods or food groups cause physical reactions. An elimination diet is a technique that uses a very specific diet of limited foods that you can eat and other foods that you must avoid. An improvement of physical symptoms is one step in determining any type of allergy problems. The eliminated or suspected foods are then carefully reintroduced in a special format and observations are made. The main goal is an adequate diet with as few restricted foods as possible.

Laboratory testing may include a skin-prick test, which uses small amounts of diluted food extracts that are scratched into the skin. If the skin reacts with a small red bump, you may have an allergy to that food. Blood tests can also be performed to check for certain antibodies that are involved with the food allergy.

Another test that may be completed in the doctor's office is a challenge test, which helps to determine whether a food can begin to be included in the diet again. In this test, the doctor gives the patient a sample of either the suspected food or a placebo. The placebo will not cause an allergic reaction. The response is carefully monitored, and if no symptoms appear, the challenge is repeated with a higher dose. For safety, this test must be completed only under a doctor's supervision.

Treatment

Once diagnosed, the only way to treat a food allergy is complete elimination of the offending food. In about a third of people with food allergies, the complete removal of an offending food from the diet for at least one to two years has been shown to eliminate the food allergy. If a food allergy forces you to eliminate an entire food group, your diet may end up lacking in some essential nutrients.

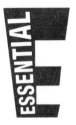

It is best not to assume that taking a supplement will take the place of a missing food group. Instead, seek out the advice of a registered dietitian, and let him or her guide you on nutritionally adequate foods to substitute for the foods you have to avoid.

Managing food allergies requires extensive knowledge of food labels, ingredient lists, and restaurant menus. You may need to contact food manufacturers for current ingredients or for answers to your questions on certain food products. Certain wording on labels or on ingredient lists can be a warning sign about the presence of a certain food. Be aware of foods that are used as ingredients in other foods, such as eggs in mayonnaise, some salad dressings, or various salads.

See Appendix C for terms for common food allergens.

Lactose Intolerance

Don't confuse lactose intolerance with a milk allergy. Being lactose intolerant means you have an intolerance to the sugar in milk (lactose) because your body does not produce enough of the enzyme lactase, which is responsible for the digestion of lactose. Left undigested, lactose can cause uncomfortable symptoms such as nausea, cramping, bloating, abdominal pain, gas, and diarrhea.

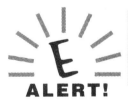

For people with a true milk allergy, it is the protein found in the milk that they are actually allergic to. People who have a true milk allergy must avoid all milk products.

Lactose intolerance can affect people in varying degrees, with some having more severe symptoms and others being able to consume more lactose. Symptoms can begin anywhere from fifteen minutes up to several hours after consuming food or a drink containing lactose. To help deal with lactose intolerance, follow some of these basic guidelines:

- Look for label ingredient terms that suggest lactose is present, such as the following: milk, dry milk solids, nonfat milk solids, buttermilk, lactose, malted milk, sour or sweet cream, margarine, milk chocolate, whey, whey protein concentrate, and cheese.
- If your intolerance is severe, it is vital to recognize baked and processed food products that might contain lactose, such as these: pancakes, biscuits, cookies, cakes, salad dressings, commercial sauces or gravies, cream soups, lunchmeats, whipped toppings, and powdered coffee creamers.
- Look for lactose-reduced or lactose-free milk products.
- Try special tablets and drops that you can add to regular milk. They will help almost completely break down the lactose after about twenty-four hours.
- Experiment so you know what you can tolerate. Start with small amounts, and gradually increase the portion size to determine your personal tolerance level.
- Consume lactose-containing foods as part of a meal instead of alone. This can sometimes make the lactose easier to digest.
- Eat smaller portions of lactose-containing foods. For example, instead of drinking a whole glass of milk, just try half of a serving.
- Choose calcium-rich foods that are naturally low in lactose, such as aged cheeses like Swiss, Colby, Parmesan, or Cheddar.
- Try yogurt for a dairy food. Many people who are lactose intolerant can tolerate yogurt because of its "friendly" bacteria to help digest the lactose.
- Don't forget about other calcium-rich foods besides dairy products, including dark green leafy vegetables, calcium-fortified products such as orange juice, and canned sardines or salmon with bones.
- Look for kosher foods that have the words "parev" or "parve" on the label. This means they are milk-free.

If you suspect lactose intolerance, do not self-diagnose. This condition can be linked to other health issues.

Celiac Disease

Celiac disease is a type of food-related condition and is often a lifelong condition. It is also known as gluten intolerance, non-tropical sprue, or gluten-sensitive enteropathy. This condition can occur at any age and is much more common than once thought. Celiac disease is an intestinal disorder in which gluten, a natural protein commonly found in many grains, including wheat, barley, rye, and oats, cannot be tolerated by the body.

When gluten is metabolized in the body, it breaks down into glutenin and gliadin, and it is actually the gliadin that does the damage for people with celiac disease. When they consume foods with gluten or gliadin, the immune system responds by damaging the villi or the walls of the small intestines that are used to help absorb nutrients. The result is that the intestine cannot absorb nutrients properly, and the person can become malnourished. Celiac disease is known as an autoimmune disease because the immune system is actually causing the damage.

Symptoms

Celiac disease can affect people differently, and symptoms and severity can vary. Some common symptoms include the following:

- Chronic diarrhea that does not get better with medication
- Foul-smelling, greasy, pale stool
- Gassiness
- Recurring abdominal bloating
- Weight loss
- Fatigue
- Infertility, lack of menstruation
- Bone or joint pain
- Depression, irritability, or mood changes

- Neurological problems, including weakness, poor balance, seizures, headaches, or numbness or tingling in the legs
- Itchy, painful skin rash
- Tooth discoloration or loss of enamel, sores on lips or tongue
- Other signs of vitamin deficiency, such as scaly skin or hyperkeratosis (from lack of vitamin A), or bleeding gums or bruising easily (from lack of vitamin K)

Treatment

Celiac disease is a genetic disorder, so there is nothing you can do to prevent it. A person with the disorder must follow a gluten-restricted, gliadin-free diet for life for successful management of the condition. Once gliadin is eliminated from the diet, the small intestines can begin to heal, nutrient absorption will improve, and symptoms will begin to disappear.

To eliminate gliadin from the diet, any foods or food components with the following four grains must be completely eliminated: wheat, rye, barley, and oats. Avoiding wheat can be a very big dietary challenge because wheat is the main ingredient in so many different foods.

To help deal with gluten intolerance, follow some of these guidelines:

- Consult a registered dietitian for information, education, and help on eating a gliadin-free diet.
- Look for gluten-free grains and other food products at specialty stores or on the Internet.
- Read food labels carefully, and become familiar with the lingo that can mean the presence of gliadin. A dietitian can help you with this.
- Become educated on the origin and composition of ingredients. For example, vinegar may seem harmless, but it actually is often distilled from a grain with gliadin and would not be appropriate if you have gluten intolerance. You would need to look for rice vinegar, wine vinegar, or pure cider vinegar.
- Use gliadin-free flour in place of wheat or white flour when cooking or baking. These types of flours include corn, rice, soy, arrowroot,

tapioca, or potato flours. They are a bit different than wheat flour, so it may take some experimentation.

- When eating away from home, make sure to ask questions when necessary or pack your own gluten-free foods when traveling on the road.
- Contact food manufacturers for current information on their ingredient lists. These are constantly changing, so you need to stay up-to-date.
- Seek out local and national support groups. These groups can be a great way to share information with people with your same condition. A registered dietitian or the Internet can help you find these types of groups.

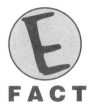

FACT

According to the National Institute of Health, an estimated 1 in 4,700 Americans have been diagnosed with celiac disease. However, it may be much more common than this. Celiac disease is the most common genetic disease in Europe.

It is vital to know the difference between gluten and gliadin when checking food labels or asking for ingredient information from manufacturers. These terms may indicate that a food contains gliadin:

- Flour, self-rising flour, enriched flour
- Modified food starch
- Monosodium glutamate (MSG)
- Hydrolyzed vegetable protein (HVP)
- Cereals
- Malt or cereal extracts
- Malt flavoring
- Distilled vinegar
- Emulsifiers
- Stabilizers
- Wheat starch

Keep in mind that the information given in this section only skims the surface of vital information you need to manage this condition. Seeking the help of a doctor and dietitian is essential for receiving *all* of the necessary information you need. If you think you may have gluten intolerance, do not self-diagnose. Consult your doctor immediately. See Appendix D for more help and information on celiac disease.

Irritable Bowel Syndrome

Irritable bowel syndrome (IBS) is a common but poorly understood disorder that can cause a variety of bowel symptoms. Symptoms of this disorder can mirror the symptoms of a number of other digestive disorders, so IBS is usually only diagnosed after your doctor has ruled out more serious possibilities. People with IBS can experience mild to severe bowel problems. For some, IBS affects everyday life.

Symptoms

Symptoms and severity of symptoms will vary among different people. People with IBS may have some or all of the following symptoms:

- Abdominal pain, discomfort, or cramping, usually relieved after a bowel movement; pain can be mild or severe.
- Periods of diarrhea, constipation, or alternating diarrhea and constipation.
- Bloating, gassiness, or a feeling of having a distended abdomen.
- Mucus in bowel movements.
- Feeling as though a bowel movement is incomplete.
- In extreme cases, nausea, dizziness, or fainting along with the other symptoms.

Treatment

One of the easiest ways to treat IBS is to change your diet to help reduce the likelihood that an IBS attack will occur. Everybody has different trigger foods. Physicians recommend keeping a food diary and tracking what you ate before attacks. After you discover your particular trigger foods, you can eliminate them from your diet. Some common IBS trigger foods include these:

- Cabbage, broccoli, kale, legumes, and other gas-producing foods
- Caffeine
- Alcohol
- Dairy products
- Fatty foods, including whole milk, cream, cheese, butter, oils, meats, and avocados

- Raw fruits
- Foods, gums, and beverages containing the sugar alcohol sorbitol

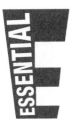

Another treatment method that may help is eating smaller meals more often versus large meals just a few times per day. Slowing down your eating may also help because eating quickly makes you swallow air, which produces belching and/or flatulence.

If constipation and abdominal pain are your main symptoms, adding fiber to your diet can help relieve this discomfort. Too much fiber at once, especially if you are not used to a higher fiber diet, can increase gas in your system, so it is important to add fiber gradually and drink plenty of water. Over time, your body will adjust to the higher intake of fiber, and the gassiness should decrease. Good sources of fiber include fresh fruit, vegetables, nuts and seeds, and whole-grain breads and cereals. Your doctor may also recommend a fiber supplement.

If symptoms are not relieved after eliminating trigger foods and adding fiber, your doctor may prescribe medications.

The Cancer Connection

Cancer is the second leading cause of death in the United States. According to the National Cancer Institute, diet and lifestyle have a definite role in preventing cancer: "Scientists estimate that as many as 50 to 75 percent of cancer deaths in the United States are caused by human behaviors such as smoking and dietary choices."

The following behaviors can help prevent cancer:

- Not using cigarettes or other tobacco products
- Not drinking too much alcohol
- Eating five or more daily servings of fruits and vegetables
- Eating a low-fat diet
- Maintaining or reaching a healthy weight
- Being physically active
- Protecting skin from sunlight

Cancer Prevention Diet

Following a healthy diet may help prevent some types of cancers. Following a healthy diet includes eating a balanced diet from all of the food groups each day.

You should aim to eat at least five servings of fruits and vegetables each day. Certain fruits and vegetables may help protect against certain cancers, such as lung cancer, because they contain "phytochemicals," or plant chemicals, and beta-carotene, a powerful antioxidant vitamin, that both seem to have cancer-fighting properties. Fruits and vegetables that are dark green, orange, red, or yellow are higher in beta-carotene. Citrus fruits and other fruits and vegetables that are high in vitamin C, another powerful antioxidant, may help to decrease the risk of esophageal and stomach cancer. Foods high in vitamin C include the following:

- Broccoli
- Cantaloupe
- Grapefruit
- Green peppers
- Kiwi fruits

- Oranges
- Potatoes (with skin)
- Strawberries
- Tangerines

Members of the cabbage family, known as cruciferous vegetables, may help decrease the risk of colon and stomach cancer. Cruciferous vegetables contain plant chemicals known as indoles, which are thought to act as natural cancer-fighters. Tomatoes and tomato-based foods contain the cancer-fighting substance lycopene. Lycopene has been shown to specifically lower the risk of cervical, colon, and prostate cancer.

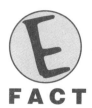

FACT

Recent research has demonstrated that regularly eating soy foods may help decrease the risk of breast and prostate cancer. Isoflavones are substances in soy foods that may have cancer-fighting as well as other healthful properties.

Both whole grains and legumes contain nutrients that may help protect against cancer such as colon cancer. Whole grains should be chosen more often than refined grains. Whole grains are richer in fiber, vitamins, and minerals than refined grains. Legumes, or dried beans and peas, should be eaten at least three times each week. Legumes are also an ideal low-fat, high-protein substitute for high-fat meats. Fruits, vegetables, legumes, and whole grains are good sources of fiber, which seems to also play an important role in the prevention of certain types of cancer.

It is recommended that fat be reduced to 15 to 30 percent of a day's total calories. To help cut back on fat, decrease your use of butter, margarine, fried foods, and rich desserts. Stick with the healthier fats or the unsaturated fats, monounsaturated and polyunsaturated. These fats can be found in vegetable oil, nuts, and seeds. Keep in mind that too much total fat, whether saturated or unsaturated, may increase the risk of breast, colon, and prostate cancer. High-fat diets may lead to obesity, which has been linked to breast, colon, gallbladder, and uterine cancer.

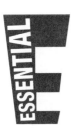

Flaxseed is a good source of the essential fatty acid omega-3 and is also a good source of fiber. Flaxseed is an abundant source of lignans, which may help to protect against hormone-sensitive cancers such as breast cancer. In moderate amounts, flaxseed can be a smart addition to your everyday diet.

Aim to consume at least two servings of low-fat or fat-free dairy products each day. Good choices are low-fat or fat-free milk and low-fat yogurt. Calcium-rich foods may help protect against colon cancer.

Alcohol should be limited to fewer than two drinks a day for men and one a day for women. Experts conclude that alcohol may increase the risk for esophageal, colon, liver, and mouth cancer. Alcohol may also increase the risk of breast cancer for women. The risk for several types of these cancers is multiplied in people who both drink and smoke.

Certain teas, including black and green, contain substances called flavonoids that may help prevent colon, esophageal, skin, and stomach cancers. So you may want to think about switching from coffee to tea once in a while.

Limiting Meat Consumption

Meat consumption should be limited, especially meats high in fat. Leaner choices of protein include skinless white-meat poultry, legumes, soy foods, and fish. It is recommended to consume fish at least once to twice per week. Fish contains polyunsaturated fats known as omega-3 essential fatty acids, which may help protect against breast, colon, esophageal, pancreatic, and stomach cancer.

Consuming too much red meat may be linked to an increased risk of colon, breast, kidney, pancreas, and prostate cancer. In the United States, red meat is a major source of saturated fat, which may actually be a separate risk factor for certain types of cancers. If you eat red meat, limit it to no more than 3 ounces per day, and choose the leanest cuts.

Limit or eliminate cured meats, which include food such as bacon, ham, hot dogs, and sausage. Salt-cured, smoked, and grilled (charred) foods may increase the risk of stomach cancer.

Diet and activity is a major risk factor of cancer that individuals can control. It only takes small changes in your everyday lifestyle to possibly prevent cancer and help you live a longer and healthier life.

Hypertension and Diet

Hypertension is another name for high blood pressure. People can have high blood pressure for years without knowing it. Left untreated, high blood pressure can contribute to many health conditions, including heart attack, stroke, heart failure, and/or kidney failure. High blood pressure is defined as a reading of 140 over 90 ml/Hg or greater.

According to current estimates, one in four U.S. adults has high blood pressure, but because there are usually no symptoms, nearly a third of these people don't even know they have it. This is why high blood pressure is often called the silent killer.

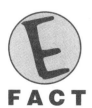

FACT

High blood pressure (hypertension) killed 42,997 Americans in 1999 and contributed to the deaths of about 227,000. As many as 50 million Americans aged six and older have high blood pressure.

Risk Factors

It is difficult to instruct people how to prevent hypertension because health experts don't yet fully understand why most cases occur. However, they do know that several lifestyle factors do contribute to high blood pressure.

Some of these are risk factors you can control, and others are not. Controllable risk factors include the following:

- **Obesity:** People with a body mass index (BMI) of 30.0 or higher are more likely to develop high blood pressure.
- **Eating too much salt:** This increases blood pressure in some people who are salt-sensitive.
- **Alcohol:** Heavy and regular use of alcohol can increase blood pressure dramatically.
- **Lack of exercise:** Being physically inactive makes it more likely that one will become overweight, which increases the risk of high blood pressure. Also, regular exercise keeps the blood flowing and the heart pumping; the heart is a muscle that needs to be strengthened, just like any other muscle in the body.
- **Stress:** This is often mentioned as a risk factor. However, stress levels vary greatly from person to person, which makes it hard to measure, and people also handle stress differently.

Uncontrollable risk factors include the following:

- **Race:** For uncertain reasons, African-Americans seem to develop high blood pressure more often than Caucasians. For African-Americans who do have high blood pressure, it tends to occur at an earlier age and is more severe.
- **Heredity:** The tendency toward high blood pressure runs in families. If someone in your immediate family has it, especially a parent, you are more likely to develop it.
- **Age:** In general, the older you get, the higher your risk for high blood pressure. It is more common in people over thirty-five. Men seem to develop it most often between thirty-five and fifty-five. Women are more likely to develop it after menopause.

Controlling Hypertension

High blood pressure is a condition that is not curable and needs to be managed for life. Your first step should be to have your blood pressure checked. If it is normal, you should continue to get it checked at least every two years. If your blood pressure is near the top of the normal range, and/or if you have a family history of high blood pressure, you are considered at high risk. If you are at high risk, your doctor will work with you on a schedule to have your blood pressure checked regularly.

If you do have high blood pressure, there are steps you should take to help reduce and control it. Your first step in managing your blood pressure is to control the risk factors that you have control over. Your doctor may include in your treatment things like weight loss, more physical activity, and a low-fat and low-sodium diet. Your doctor may also highly recommend that you quit smoking, if you are a smoker, to help reduce your overall risk for stroke and heart attack.

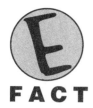

FACT

Less active, less fit people have a 30- to 50-percent greater risk for developing high blood pressure.

Reducing your alcohol intake may also be recommended. Depending on the severity of your condition, a prescription medication may be given to help you control your blood pressure. Both doctors and patients usually prefer to control blood pressure with lifestyle changes first, but often antihypertensive medication is needed to provide adequate control. Your doctor will be the one to decide what your treatment should be but make sure you are involved in every aspect.

If you don't have high blood pressure, it is still important to control the risk factors that can put you at risk in the future.

Taking Care of Your Heart

Heart disease is the leading killer of Americans today. Several risk factors are known to directly contribute to a higher risk of heart disease for both men and women; the more factors a person exhibits, the greater the risk.

Risk factors include:

- Elevated cholesterol, especially with elevated LDL and low HDL
- Elevated triglycerides
- Smoking
- High blood pressure
- Diabetes
- Sedentary lifestyle
- Obesity, especially when the fat is concentrated above the waist area
- Stress
- Family history of heart disease
- Gender and age (risk starts earlier for men, increases for women postmenopause)

You can reduce your risk by controlling all heart disease risk factors listed, except of course for family history, gender, and age. Your doctor can help you assess your overall risk, but common sense should tell you to improve your lifestyle by eating healthier, exercising, and avoiding all forms of tobacco as well as secondhand smoke when possible.

Several nutritional factors are important in helping to prevent heart disease. To reduce the impact of the controllable risk factors for heart disease, the American Heart Association (AHA) recommends the following population-wide dietary and lifestyle goals:

- Eliminate cigarette smoking
- Consume appropriate level of calories and perform physical activity to prevent obesity and reduce weight in those who are overweight
- Consume 30 percent or fewer of the day's total calories from fat
- Consume 8 to 10 percent of total calories from saturated fat
- Consume up to 10 percent of total calories from polyunsaturated fat
- Consume up to 15 percent of total calories from monounsaturated fat
- Consume less than 300 mg of cholesterol daily
- Consume no more than 2,400 mg of sodium daily
- Consume 55 to 60 percent of calories as complex carbohydrates
- For those who drink and those for whom alcohol is not contraindicated, consumption should not exceed two drinks (1 to 2 ounces) per day

Other recommendations include consuming at least 25 to 30 grams of fiber each day from sources such as whole grains, fruits, vegetables, and legumes. Consuming a variety of fruits and vegetables will also ensure that you receive plenty of beta-carotene, vitamin C, folic acid, vitamin E, and other antioxidants and protective substances such as flavonoids and carotenoids. You can regularly add foods such as soy, oat bran, fish, nuts, seeds, and garlic to strengthen your disease-fighting prevention diet even more.

You are also advised to talk to your doctor about your risk for heart disease and how to manage any risk factors you may have.

Diabetes

In the United States, approximately 17 million people have diabetes. Diabetes is a disease that prevents the body from producing or properly using insulin. Insulin is a hormone that the body needs to convert sugar, starches, and other food into energy needed for daily life. In healthy people, insulin helps regulate blood sugar levels. People with diabetes have trouble controlling blood sugar.

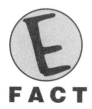

FACT

Today, the incidence of Type 2 diabetes is nearing epidemic proportions. This is in large part due to the increased number of older Americans, the increased rate of obesity, and the increase in sedentary lifestyles of Americans.

There are two major types of diabetes. In **Type 1** diabetes, the body does not produce any insulin. This type most often occurs in children and young adults, but not always. People with Type 1 diabetes must take a daily injection of insulin to survive. Type 1 diabetes accounts for 5 to 10 percent of diabetes.

In **Type 2** diabetes, the body does not make enough insulin or use it properly. It is the most common form of the disease. Type 2 diabetes accounts for 90 to 95 percent of all people with diabetes. Obesity is a major risk factor for developing Type 2 diabetes.

Complications

There are many complications associated with diabetes, and most are strongly related to high blood sugar levels. In fact, with its complications, diabetes is the seventh leading cause of death in the United States. It is estimated that each year, at least 190,000 people die as a result of diabetes and its complications. Keeping your blood sugar levels in your target range is your best defense against the complications of diabetes.

Complications can include the following:

- Blindness
- Kidney disease
- Gum disease
- Skin disorders

- Heart disease and stroke
- Nerve disease and amputations
- Impotence

To lower your risk of these complications, get regular check-ups, be aware of warning signs, keep blood sugar levels close to normal, control your weight, eat a healthy, well-balanced diet, get regular exercise, check your feet every day for minor cuts or blisters and show them to your health-care practitioner, and do not smoke.

Symptoms

For some, diabetes can go undiagnosed because some of the symptoms seem so mild and/or harmless. Recent studies indicate that early detection and treatment is the key to decreasing the complications of diabetes later on.

Some of the symptoms of diabetes may include the following:

- Frequent urination
- Excessive thirst
- Extreme hunger
- Unusual weight loss

- Increased fatigue
- Irritability
- Blurry vision

If you have one or more of these symptoms, you should see your doctor immediately.

Managing Diabetes with Diet

Managing diabetes with diet means eating well-balanced, healthy meals. Along with nutrition, other lifestyle modifications such as exercise, a healthy weight, and medications (insulin or oral diabetes pills) are essential to good diabetes control. Controlling diabetes means keeping blood sugar levels as close to normal (non-diabetic level) as possible.

In the past, strict diets for diabetics were used, but more recently they have become more flexible. Following a "diabetic diet" is really no different from that of a typical healthy diet for a person without diabetes. Diabetics should limit fat, sodium, and sugar intake as well as get plenty of fruits, vegetables, whole grains, and fat-free or low-fat dairy products.

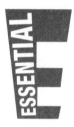

It is important to work closely with a registered dietitian to design a meal plan that is right for you—one that fits into your lifestyle and includes foods that you enjoy. A diabetic meal plan acts as a guide to show you how much and what types of foods you should choose for meals and snacks.

Fiber is an important part of a healthy diet and can also be helpful in controlling blood sugar levels. The soluble type of fiber from legumes, oats, fruits, and some vegetables may help slow the rate at which blood sugar is absorbed into the bloodstream. This can keep blood sugar levels from rising rapidly.

The main goal is to choose a plan that will help the person to control his or her blood sugar levels. It is important that diabetics learn how to self-manage their condition as well as their diet.

Management of the diet for a Type 1 diabetic is to coordinate food intake with the action of the insulin they are using. Management of the diet in a Type 2 diabetic is to restrict calories for weight loss, educate for better food choices, and spread foods throughout the day. Weight loss of 10 to 20 pounds has been shown to reduce high blood sugar levels. Spreading meals out throughout the day may be beneficial by helping to keep insulin and blood sugar levels more stable.

With treatment, blood sugar levels may go down to normal again. But this does not mean a diabetic is cured. Instead, a blood sugar level in the target range shows that the treatment plan is working and that the diabetes is being managed correctly.

Exercise

Exercise, along with good nutrition and medication, is also important for good diabetes control. Increasing activity helps the body transport glucose to the body's cells. It also helps lower blood sugar levels and helps reduce the risk for heart disease and obesity. Exercise usually lowers blood sugar, which helps your body use its food supply better. Also, exercise may help insulin work better. Your health-care provider can help you decide what kinds of exercise and how much exercise are best suited to your needs. If your blood sugar control is poor, do not exercise. Get medical advice first.

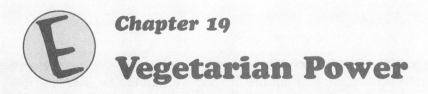

Chapter 19

Vegetarian Power

People have many reasons—ethical, religious, environmental, personal, and health concerns among them—for choosing a vegetarian lifestyle. For some, vegetarianism is strictly a way of eating, while for others it is a way of life. A plant-based diet that is based on a wide variety of foods can be a healthy choice.

Being a Vegetarian

Vegetarian is defined as eating no meat, poultry, or fish. Though it is a matter of personal choice, some vegetarians avoid all animal products. Others may consume eggs and/or dairy products. Only a small percentage of vegetarians are actually strict vegetarians who avoid all animal products.

Vegetarians can be classified into several different categories:

- **Vegan or strict vegetarian:** consumes absolutely no animal foods, including foods with animal product as ingredients. These are the strictest types of vegetarians.
- **Lacto-vegetarian:** consumes dairy foods but no other animal foods including eggs.
- **Lacto-ovo-vegetarian:** consumes dairy foods plus eggs, but no other animal foods.
- **Semi-vegetarian:** mostly follows a vegetarian diet (lacto-ovo-vegetarian), but consumes meat, poultry, and fish occasionally.

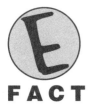

FACT

Vegetarianism has grown substantially in the United States in the last decade. It has become common to find meat substitutes in major grocery stores—not just health food stores. And veggie options in restaurants have also become more common.

Health Advantages

If planned properly, vegetarian diets tend to be healthier than diets that include animal foods. However, these diets can cause nutritional imbalances if not planned correctly. A healthy, well-planned vegetarian diet contains more fiber and is lower in fat, especially saturated fat, and cholesterol. It also tends to be lower in calories and higher in certain vitamins and minerals. Vegetarian diets can offer additional disease protection benefits due to their lower saturated fat, cholesterol, and animal protein content. Also, the often higher content of folate, antioxidants such as vitamin C and E, carotenoids, and phytochemicals give these diets an extra disease-fighting punch.

The incidence of death from heart disease is lower in vegetarians. Total cholesterol and LDL cholesterol (the "bad" cholesterol) levels are also usually lower. Vegetarians also tend to have a lower incidence of hypertension, Type 2 diabetes, obesity, and some forms of cancers such as lung and colon than nonvegetarians. However, not properly balancing a vegetarian diet will not result in these lower incidences.

Vegetarian Menu Planning

Vegetarian eating can supply your body with all of its needed nutrients if the menu is planned correctly. Taking the correct menu-planning approaches is vital to a diet full of adequate nutrition. The following guidelines can help vegetarians plan a healthful diet:

- Choose a variety of foods, including whole grains, vegetables, fruits, legumes, nuts, seeds, and, if desired, low-fat or fat-free dairy products and eggs.
- Choose whole, unrefined foods more often and minimize your intake of highly sweetened, fatty, and heavily refined foods.
- Choose a variety of fruits and vegetables.
- If animal foods such as dairy products and eggs are used, choose lower-fat versions of these foods. Limit cheese, other high-fat dairy foods, and eggs that are high in saturated fat.
- Vegans or strict vegetarians should make sure to include a regular source of vitamin B_{12} in their diets. Also important is vitamin D, especially if sun exposure is limited.
- Breastfed vegan infants should have vitamin B_{12} supplements if the mother's diet is not fortified.
- Be careful not to restrict dietary fat in children under two years of age. For older children, include some foods higher in unsaturated fats (such as nuts, seeds, peanut butter, avocados, and vegetable oils) to help meet nutrient and energy needs.

The Vegetarian Food Guide Pyramid is very similar to that of the regular Food Guide Pyramid. The vegetarian version provides recommended guidelines for the vegetarian population.

Table 19-1 Food Guide Pyramid for Vegetarian Meal Planning		
Food group	Daily Servings	Sample Servings
Fats, oils, and sweets	Use sparingly	Candy, butter, margarine, salad dressing, cooking oil
Milk, yogurt, and cheese group	0–3 servings daily*	1 cup milk, 1 cup yogurt, 1½ ounces natural cheese
Dried beans, nuts, seeds, eggs,and meat-substitutes group	2–3 servings daily	1 cup soy milk, ½ cup cooked dry beans or peas, 1 egg or 2 egg whites, 2 tablespoons nuts or seeds, ¼ cup tofu or tempeh, 2 tablespoons peanut butter
Vegetable group	3–5 servings daily	½ cup cooked or chopped raw vegetables, 1 cup raw leafy vegetables
Fruit group	2–4 servings daily	¾ cup juice, ¼ cup dried fruit, ½ cup chopped, raw fruit, ½ cup canned fruit, 1 medium-size piece of fruit, such as banana, apple, or orange
Bread, cereal, rice, and pasta group**	6–11 servings daily	1 slice bread, ½ bagel, 1 ounce ready-to-eat cereal, ½ cup cooked cereal, ½ cup cooked rice, pasta, or other grains

*Vegetarians who choose not to use milk, yogurt, or cheese should select other foods rich in calcium.
**Choose whole-wheat and whole-grain more often.

Nutritional Considerations

Without animal foods in the diet, several nutrients may come up short. Nutrients that should be given special attention include vitamin B_{12}, vitamin D, calcium, iron, and zinc. Careful planning can ensure the intake of all these essential nutrients each day.

Vitamin B_{12} is a nutritional concern for vegetarians because plants are not a good source of this vitamin. Consuming foods fortified with vitamin B_{12}, such as fortified breakfast cereals, soy-milk products, or vegetarian burgers, is advised for vegetarians who avoid or limit animal foods. You may also need to consider a supplement. If you do choose a supplement, do not take more than 100 percent of the RDA. When reading labels, look for the word "cyanocobalamin," the form of vitamin B_{12} best absorbed by the body.

Deficiency symptoms of vitamin B_{12} can be delayed for some time because the requirements are so small and because the vitamin is both stored and recycled in the body. The absorption of vitamin B_{12} slows down as a person ages, so supplements may be advised for older vegetarians.

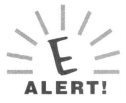

ALERT!

Be aware that spirulina, algae, seaweed, tempeh, and miso are not good sources of vitamin B_{12} even though the label says they are. The B_{12} in these products is not in a form that the body can use efficiently.

Vitamin D is still another vitamin of concern for vegetarians. This vitamin is not an issue if you drink milk and are exposed to plenty of sunlight. The body makes vitamin D on its own when your skin is exposed to sunlight. Vegans who do not consume any dairy products need to be careful to get enough vitamin D. Vitamin D can be obtained from fortified foods such as breakfast cereals, soy milk, and supplements.

One of calcium's most important functions is to keep our bones strong and healthy. If you drink milk and consume other dairy products, you do not need to worry about calcium intake. If you do not, it is important to concentrate on getting calcium in other foods. Foods other than dairy that contain calcium include legumes or dried beans, tofu, tempeh, textured vegetable protein, fortified soy milk, soy nuts, collards, broccoli, kale, spinach, rhubarb, bok choy, turnip greens, calcium-fortified orange juice, calcium-fortified grains and cereals, dried figs, nuts, seeds, salmon (with bones), and sardines (with bones).

Iron often comes up short whether you are vegetarian or not. Although vegetarian diets are usually higher in total iron content than nonvegetarian diets, iron stores are lower in vegetarians because the iron from plant foods is poorly absorbed. Plant foods provide some iron in the form of nonheme iron, which is not absorbed in the body as well as iron from animal foods, which is called heme iron. The challenge for vegetarians is to improve the absorption of the nonheme iron that they consume from plants. Following some of these guidelines will help:

- Consume plant sources that contain iron, including legumes, iron-fortified cereals and breads (especially whole-grain or whole-wheat), tofu, some dark green leafy vegetables (such as spinach and beet greens), seeds, prune juice, and dried fruit.
- Include a vitamin C–rich food at every meal, which will help your body absorb the nonheme iron from plant sources. Vitamin C–rich foods include citrus fruits, citrus juices, broccoli, tomatoes, and green pepper.
- If you are a semivegetarian, eat a small amount of meat, poultry, or fish with plant foods to help the nonheme iron absorb better.

Zinc is a mineral that is important for growth, repairing body cells, and energy products. Zinc is not widely available in plant foods, so vegetarians may come up short. Lacto-ovo vegetarians can get zinc from milk, cheese, yogurt, and eggs. For vegans, some plant foods contain zinc but in amounts less than what is found in animal foods. The key is to eat larger amounts of zinc-containing plant foods. For vegans to get enough zinc, it is also important to eat a variety of plant foods with zinc, such as whole-wheat bread, whole grains, wheat germ, bran, legumes, tofu, seeds, and nuts.

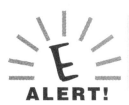

ALERT!

If you take a zinc supplement, be cautious of high doses, which can have harmful side effects. Stick with a multivitamin that provides no more than 100 percent of the RDA.

The body absorbs less zinc from plant sources because phytic acid, a substance in fiber, combines with zinc and prevents it from being fully absorbed. Therefore, to meet the RDA, it is extremely important for strict vegetarians to get plenty of zinc-containing plant foods.

Protein

Protein is a vital part of a healthy diet. The concern of enough protein intake usually surfaces with vegetarians because they do not eat most animal products and those are the most concentrated sources of complete proteins.

Plant foods contain protein and essential amino acids, but they do not contain all of the nine necessary for creating complete proteins. However, a vegetarian diet can very easily provide adequate amounts of these amino acids if a variety of plant foods are consumed daily and caloric intake is sufficient.

In the past it was recommended that vegetarians eat certain combinations of plant foods to ensure they received complete proteins at each meal. Experts now agree that there is no need to combine specific foods at meals as long as throughout the day a vegetarian concentrates on consuming various sources of amino acids. This should ensure adequate essential amino acid intake needed to build protein. A varied diet of beans, lentils, grains, and vegetables contains all of the essential amino acids your body needs.

Vegetarian Throughout the Life Cycle

During pregnancy and breastfeeding, your need for all nutrients increases. For example, you need more calcium, folic acid, and protein. If you have already mastered the concept of healthy vegetarian eating, you should be able to easily provide the nourishment you need for a healthy, full-term pregnancy. If you are new to the concept, it is important to seek the guidance of a dietitian to help you plan appropriately. As with all vegetarians, it is important to make sure you are getting plenty of calcium, vitamin D, vitamin B_{12}, iron, and protein.

During breastfeeding, remember that you need more calories than you did while pregnant. Breastfeeding women need to make sure they are consuming plenty of vitamin B_{12} sources because intake can affect levels in the breast milk. If you are concerned about nutrient intake, consult your doctor about supplements.

If your child or teenager follows a vegetarian diet, it is extremely important to monitor their intake and to consult a dietitian or your doctor for support and nutritional counseling. For vegans, there may be a need for supplements.

Becoming a Vegetarian

If you are already a vegetarian, make sure your diet is providing you with all of your needed nutrients. If you are considering becoming a vegetarian, you now know some of the basics. Here are a few more guidelines to get you started:

- Explore new foods at your grocery store. Pick out a different meat-free or soy product from the variety located in the freezer section or the health section to try at home each week. Many grocery stores now have special soy sections.
- Try something easy like topping your next pizza with a mountain of veggies and no meats. Get really brave and leave off the cheese, too.
- Use cooked legumes instead of meat in casseroles, stews, soups, and chili.
- Try some of your favorite meat dishes with a soy substitute such as textured vegetable protein instead of ground meat in Sloppy Joes or cubed tofu in a stir-fry instead of chicken.
- Load up on fresh fruits and vegetables. If you get a snack attack, grab a piece of fruit or keep cut-up fresh veggies in the fridge.
- Next time you grill out, try a marinated portabella mushroom or veggie burger on the grill instead of a ground-beef burger.
- Buy a new cookbook or look for meatless recipes on the Internet. Try at least one new recipe each week. Before you know it, you will have tasted a ton of new recipes.
- Try a vegetarian entrée at your favorite restaurant. You may be pleasantly surprised at the number of meat-free dishes there are and how great they taste.

The Joy of Soy

Soy is rapidly becoming one of nature's super foods. Researchers are uncovering more and more about the health benefits of adding soy to the diet. They are only beginning to understand the possible potential that soy has as a nutritional source of power. You don't need to be a vegetarian to add soy to your diet and reap its healthful benefits.

Soy foods are foods that have soybeans or soy protein as their major protein ingredient. The protein found in soybeans is a complete protein. The only other foods that contain complete proteins are animal foods. Soy is the *only* plant food that contains complete proteins.

Soy's Nutritional Benefits

Unlike foods from animal sources, soy is cholesterol-free. It contains no saturated fat, is a great source of fiber, contains calcium, vitamin E, and B vitamins, and is rich in the two polyunsaturated fats essential to optimal health. Most soy foods are also high in iron and are an excellent source of protein compared to other plant sources.

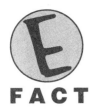

FACT

One serving of tempeh, a soy food, has more fiber than the average American consumes in an entire day.

Soybeans and the foods made from them are rich in a special compound called isoflavones. Isoflavones are the substances found in soy that are responsible for all of the health benefits that soy offers. Isoflavones are one type of a larger group of plant chemicals called phytochemicals. These plant chemicals have numerous and positive effects on human health and are found only in plant sources, especially soy.

Isoflavones are commonly referred to as "plant estrogens" because of the similar properties they have to the human hormone estrogen, though their effects are much weaker. Isoflavones in soy may help improve health in women. Recent studies have shown that isoflavones may help to lower the risk of breast cancer, though more research needs to be done before concrete statements can be made. Isoflavones have also been shown to possibly reduce some of the symptoms of menopause that women suffer. Researchers found that women who ate ½ cup of soy flour daily experienced a decline in menopausal symptoms.

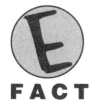

FACT

In Japan, where soy foods are a part of their everyday diet, there is no word in their language that means "hot flash." In other words Japanese women do not even know what that symptom is.

Consuming soy food can have a positive impact on bone health by helping to decrease the risk for osteoporosis. Because soy foods are rich in calcium they help increase intake and they also help to reduce calcium loss from the bones, unlike animal proteins. Isoflavones may also directly slow down the breakdown of bone mass that naturally comes with the aging process.

After menopause, women are at an increased risk for heart disease because their body begins to decrease production of estrogen, a hormone that helped protect the heart. Soy foods may help to give women extra protection against heart disease by helping to lower blood cholesterol levels, reducing cholesterol oxidation that can damage arteries, and providing isoflavones that can inhibit blood clot formation. Soy foods may help reduce the risk for heart disease for men as well as women.

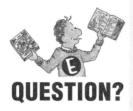

QUESTION?

Should I take a soy supplement to help decrease the risk of health problems?
At this point there is not enough concrete evidence to show a direct link between taking a soy supplement and lowering your risk of certain health problems. It is recommended instead to consume moderate amounts of soy foods as part of a healthy diet plan and not take high levels of soy in the form of supplements until more is known.

Other health benefits of soy include possibly decreasing the risk for certain types of cancers. As little as one serving of soy foods each day seems to protect against many types of cancers. Soy foods may aid in diabetes control by slowing the absorption of glucose (blood sugar) into the bloodstream and keeping blood sugar levels more steady. Soy foods may help to increase the intake of iron because they are high in this mineral. Iron deficiency can lead to anemia, which can lead to symptoms such as fatigue, headaches, and increased risk for infection. Iron deficiency is the most common nutritional problem in the world.

Soy on Food Labels

In 1999, the Food and Drug Administration (FDA) approved a new health claim that links consuming soy protein with a reduced risk of heart disease. The FDA based its approval of the health claim on several scientific studies that showed a consumption of 25 grams of soy protein per day had a cholesterol-lowering effect. The newly approved health claim can now be found on a variety of soy food labels. It reads, "25 grams of soy protein a day, as part of a diet low in saturated fat and cholesterol, may reduce the risk of heart disease. A serving of (name of food) provides _____ grams of soy protein." In order for a soy product to carry this new health claim, the food must contain at least 6.25 grams of soy protein per serving. Some examples of soy foods and their protein content include the following:

- ½ cup roasted soy nuts (12–15 grams of protein)
- 4 ounces of firm tofu (13 grams of protein)
- 1 cup of regular plain soy milk (10 grams of protein)

Soy Is Worth a Try

Eating soy foods everyday is not a guarantee against disease or any of the health problems mentioned here. Much of the research and findings to this point are speculative. But the evidence is growing that soy can positively impact the health of both men and women. Though there is presently no assurance against health problems, it is a fact that soy is an excellent source of protein, fiber, and many vitamins and minerals. As mentioned, it is also cholesterol-free, has no saturated fat, and contains the type of fat that is healthy. Adding soy to your diet can be easy as well as healthy and it is a great protein source for vegetarians.

Soy foods come in many forms, and the list is growing. Some common soy products include tofu, soy milk, tempeh, soy cheese, soy nuts, okara, veggie burgers, veggie hot dogs, soy yogurt, textured vegetable protein, and soy flour.

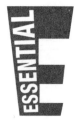

Tofu by itself is quite bland, but it does absorb the flavor of whatever ingredients it is cooked with, such as in sauces or casseroles. It can be eaten both cooked and uncooked.

Add more soy to your recipes by trying some of these substitutions:

- 1 cup dairy milk = 1 cup fortified soy milk
- 1 tablespoon margarine = ¾ tablespoon soybean oil
- 1 egg = 1 tablespoon soy flour + 1 tablespoon water or 2 ounces silken tofu
- 1 cup fruited yogurt = 1 cup soft silken tofu + blended fruit
- 1 cup ricotta cheese = 1 cup firm tofu, mashed
- Replace ½ of the cream in soup or sauces with silken tofu
- Replace ½ of the cream cheese in cheesecakes with silken tofu

Make sure you buy the right tofu for your recipe: soft/silken is good for smoothies, and firm or extra-firm is good for sautéing, baking, broiling, or stir-frying.

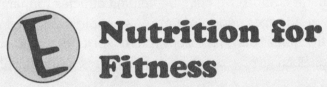

Chapter 20

Nutrition for Fitness

Whether you are a professional athlete or simply someone who loves to work out, good nutrition is a fundamental part of peak performance. No matter what sport or exercise you engage in, you can use the Food Guide Pyramid as your eating guide. To work at your best capacity is important to ensure you are consuming an overall healthy diet.

Don't Forget Your Carbs

Carbohydrates are your body's main source of energy for exercise and for everyday life. Carbohydrates should provide at least 55 to 60 percent of your overall daily calories. A person who engages in more intense endurance exercise programs will need a few more carbohydrates. Carbohydrates offer a competitive edge by helping athletes to maintain rigorous activity for a longer period of time. As people train, their body becomes more efficient at burning carbohydrates for energy and storing them in the muscles as glycogen, which is fuel that is ready for physical activity.

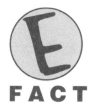

FACT

Carbohydrates provide the muscles with ongoing energy in the form of glucose and help maintain prolonged endurance and optimal performance.

The higher the intensity of an exercise, the more glycogen is used. The lower the intensity and longer the activity, the more fat is used and less glycogen.

Carbohydrates from foods include both complex or starches and sugars. Both types of carbohydrates provide energy to the body and are used to replenish muscle glycogen that is used. The biggest difference is that sugars are digested and absorbed more quickly into the bloodstream. The best source for normal training is complex carbohydrates such as whole grains, cereal, legumes, fruits, and starchy vegetables.

The muscles and the liver store glycogen (stored glucose) but only in limited amounts. Glycogen needs to be replaced after each session of exercise. Endurance athletes use a technique called "carbohydrate loading" so that they don't run out of glycogen or stored energy during a long-distance activity. They eat tons of carbohydrates to have "extra" stored glycogen on hand for extended activities. A seven-day regimen was commonly used by athletes until recently. Research now shows that three days of rest and extra complex carbohydrates is simpler and just as effective.

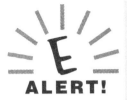

Carbohydrate loading is most effective with trained athletes. Because of training and more muscle, their bodies have a greater capacity to store extra glycogen. This technique is not recommended for children, teens, and people with diabetes or high triglycerides. People who are moderately active can store only so much glycogen in their muscles and therefore may gain weight if they practice carbo loading.

Protein Plus

Everyone needs protein, whether an athlete or not. Protein not only has many important functions in the body, it also supplies energy. However, protein is not your best choice for extra energy. Protein should supply 12 to 15 percent of your overall calorie intake. Most athletes or heavy exercisers only need slightly larger amounts of protein than sedentary people.

Protein is best figured on a personal basis by body weight and activity. Use **TABLE 20-1** to figure your protein needs—simply multiply your weight by the grams given in your category.

Table 20-1 Protein Needs Based on Activity Level	
Exercise Category	**Recommended Daily Protein Needs**
Sedentary People	0.36 grams per pound of body weight
Moderate Exercisers	0.36–0.5 grams per pound of body weight
Endurance Athletes	0.5–0.8 grams per pound of body weight
Strength Athletes	0.6–0.8 grams per pound of body weight

Protein is not what builds muscle or makes them stronger. Only exercise, especially weight training, will do that. Most people already eat too much protein, and excess can put extra stress on your kidneys and rob your body of calcium. Even serious exercise will not exhaust most people's supply of protein. Amino acid supplements also will not increase muscle size or strength.

Fluids for Peak Performance

Fluids are another important part of an athlete's overall healthy diet. Both athletes and nonathletes alike often forget about fluids and/or water intake. During any type of physical activity, your performance, endurance, and strength rely on it. When you exercise, you sweat. By sweating you are losing valuable fluids and electrolytes that must be replaced. Just losing as little as 2 to 3 percent of your body weight from fluid can hinder your performance and begin to lead to dehydration.

Fluids help in the energy production cycle and help cool your body down when it heats up from exercise. They carry other nutrients, such as electrolytes, through your bloodstream and help cushion your body's tissues and organs from the jolts of exercise.

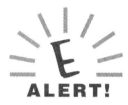

ALERT!

Never drink alcoholic beverages before or during a heavy workout. Alcohol promotes dehydration and can also impair your coordination, muscle reflexes, reaction time, and balance.

It is important to drink fluids before, during, and after exercise. Even if you don't feel thirsty, make sure you drink fluids. For workouts that are shorter than sixty minutes, water is a great choice. If working out or engaging in a physical activity that will last more than an hour, sports drinks may be a better choice. If you are exercising in very hot and humid weather, make sure you drink even more fluid.

Table 20-2 Fluid-Drinking Schedule	
When	**How Much**
2 hours prior to activity	2 cups of fluid (water, juice, milk, etc.)
Just prior to activity	2 cups of water or sports drink
Every 15 minutes during activity	½ cup water or sports drink
After activity	2 cups water or sports drink, for every pound lost during the activity until you return to your pre-exercise weight

If you are a moderate exerciser, concentrate on drinking at least 64 ounces of water per day and drink water before, during, and after your exercise routine.

Electrolytes

When you sweat you lose electrolytes, which include sodium, chloride, and potassium. One function of electrolytes is to maintain the water balance in your body. They also help muscles to contract and relax. Sodium is one of the electrolytes you lose the most of. You can most likely replace those electrolytes, including sodium, by the foods you eat in a normal diet. The average American consumes more than enough sodium to replace any lost through perspiration. Therefore there is no need for salt or sodium pills. If you perspire heavily, it is more important to concentrate on extra fluids instead. If you are an endurance athlete who perspires for long periods of time, a sports drink will probably offer enough sodium to replace what you have lost.

Energy Needs

How many calories you need each day is a very individual topic. The amount of energy you need for various sports depends on your body composition, body weight, fitness level, and the activity you participate in. For example, the more muscle you have, the more energy or calories your body burns, so the more calories you need. Also, the more intense your activity is, the more you accomplish, and the length of time you spend doing it all contribute to calculating your calorie needs. Obviously some sports burn more calories than others. To estimate your calorie needs, review Chapter 1.

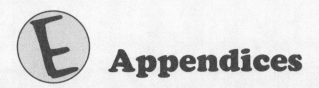 **Appendices**

Appendix A

Body Mass Index Table

Body weight (pounds)

BMI	19	20	21	22	23	24	25	26	27	28	29	30	31	32	33	34	35	36	37	38	39	40	41	42	43	44	45	46	47	48	49	50	51	52	53	54
Height (inches)																																				
58	91	96	100	105	110	115	119	124	129	134	138	143	148	153	158	162	167	172	177	181	186	191	196	201	205	210	215	220	224	229	234	239	244	248	253	258
59	94	99	104	109	114	119	124	128	133	138	143	148	153	158	163	168	173	178	183	188	193	198	203	208	212	217	222	227	232	237	242	247	252	257	262	267
60	97	102	107	112	118	123	128	133	138	143	148	153	158	163	168	174	179	184	189	194	199	204	209	215	220	225	230	235	240	245	250	255	261	266	271	276
61	100	106	111	116	122	127	132	137	143	148	153	158	164	169	174	180	185	190	195	201	206	211	217	222	227	232	238	243	248	254	259	264	269	275	280	285
62	104	109	115	120	126	131	136	142	147	153	158	164	169	175	180	186	191	196	202	207	213	218	224	229	235	240	246	251	256	262	267	273	278	284	289	295
63	107	113	118	124	130	135	141	146	152	158	163	169	175	180	186	191	197	203	208	214	220	225	231	237	242	248	254	259	265	270	278	282	287	293	299	304
64	110	116	122	128	134	140	145	151	157	163	169	174	180	186	192	197	204	209	215	221	227	232	238	244	250	256	262	267	273	279	285	291	296	302	308	314
65	114	120	126	132	138	144	150	156	162	168	174	180	186	192	198	204	210	216	222	228	234	240	246	252	258	264	270	276	282	288	294	300	306	312	318	324
66	118	124	130	136	142	148	155	161	167	173	179	186	192	198	204	210	216	223	229	235	241	247	253	260	266	272	278	284	291	297	303	309	315	322	328	334
67	121	127	134	140	146	153	159	166	172	178	185	191	198	204	211	217	223	230	236	242	249	255	261	268	274	280	287	293	299	306	312	319	325	331	338	344
68	125	131	138	144	151	158	164	171	177	184	190	197	203	210	216	223	230	236	243	249	256	262	269	276	282	289	295	302	308	315	322	328	335	341	348	354
69	128	135	142	149	155	162	169	176	182	189	196	203	209	216	223	230	236	243	250	257	263	270	277	284	291	297	304	311	318	324	331	338	345	351	358	365
70	132	139	146	153	160	167	174	181	188	195	202	209	216	222	229	236	243	250	257	264	271	278	285	292	299	306	313	320	327	334	341	348	355	362	369	376
71	136	143	150	157	165	172	179	186	193	200	208	215	222	229	236	243	250	257	265	272	279	286	293	301	308	315	322	329	338	343	351	358	365	372	379	386
72	140	147	154	162	169	177	184	191	199	206	213	221	228	235	242	250	258	265	272	279	287	294	302	309	316	324	331	338	346	353	361	368	375	383	390	397
73	144	151	159	166	174	182	189	197	204	212	219	227	235	242	250	257	265	272	280	288	295	302	310	318	325	333	340	348	355	363	371	378	386	393	401	408
74	148	155	163	171	179	186	194	202	210	218	225	233	241	249	256	264	272	280	287	295	303	311	319	326	334	342	350	358	365	373	381	389	396	404	412	420
75	152	160	168	176	184	192	200	208	216	224	232	240	248	256	264	272	279	287	295	303	311	319	327	335	343	351	359	367	375	383	391	399	407	415	423	431
76	156	164	172	180	189	197	205	213	221	230	238	246	254	263	271	279	287	295	304	312	320	328	336	344	353	361	369	377	385	394	402	410	418	426	435	443

Normal   **Overweight**   **Obese**   **Extreme Obesity**

Source: Adapted from *Clinical Guidelines on the Identification, Evaluation, and Treatment of Overweight and Obesity in Adults: The Evidence Report.*

Appendix B

Good Sources of Nutrients

Good Sources of Vitamin A

Apricots

Broccoli

Cantaloupe

Carrots

Collards

Kale

Mango

Pumpkin

Spinach

Squash, winter

Sweet potato

Tomato

Turnip greens

Watermelon

Good Sources of Vitamin C

Apple with skin

Apricot, dried

Banana

Beans, lima

Broccoli

Cantaloupe

Collards

Grapefruit

Grapefruit juice

Honeydew melon

Kale

Kiwi

Orange

Orange juice

Pear with skin

Peas, green

Peppers

Potato, with skin

Spinach

Squash, winter

Strawberries

Sweet potato

Tomato

Turnip greens

Watermelon

Good Sources of Folate

Beans, dry

Black-eyed peas

Broccoli

Lentils

Mustard greens

Orange

Orange juice

Peas, green

Peas, split

Spinach

Turnip greens

Good Sources of Potassium

Apricots, dried

Banana

Beans, dry

Black-eyed peas

Cantaloupe

Grapefruit juice

Honeydew melon

Lentils

Orange juice

Peas, green

Peas, split

Plantains

Potato

Potato with skin

Prune juice

Spinach, cooked

Squash, winter

Sweet potato

Tomato

Good Sources of Dietary Fiber

Apple with skin

Apricot, dried

Banana

Beans, dry

Beans, lima

Black-eyed peas

Broccoli

Carrots

Lentils

Orange

Pear with skin

Peas, green

Peas, split

Potato with skin

Prunes

Spinach

Squash, winter

Strawberries

Sweet potato

Tomato

Note: A good source of a vitamin or mineral contributes at least 10 percent of its Percent Daily Value per serving. A good source of dietary fiber contributes at least 2 grams of dietary fiber per serving.

Appendix C

Terms for Common Allergens

Check labels and ingredient lists for the following words, which indicate the presence of a particular allergen.

Allergen	Ingredient Term	Allergen	Ingredient Term
Milk	Milk	**Egg**	Albumin
	Buttermilk		Dried egg solids
	Casein		Egg white
	Caseinate		Globulin
	Cheese		Livetin
	Cottage cheese		Ovalbumin
	Cream		Ovoglobulin
	Curds		Ovomucin
	Ghee		Ovomucoid
	Ice cream	**Ovovitellin**	Vitellin
	Nonfat milk solids	**Corn**	Fresh, canned, or creamed corn
	Whey		Cornmeal
	Yogurt		Hominy or corn grits
Casein Hydrolysate	Sodium caseinate		Maize
	Dried milk solids	**Popcorn/corn solids**	Cornstarch
	Lactate solids		Baking powder (unless corn-free)
	Lactoalbumin		Corn syrup
	Lactoglobulin		Dextrose
	Milk solid pastes		Vegetable gum
	Sweetened condensed milk		Vegetable starch
	Whey or whey solids		

Allergen	Ingredient Term
Dextrin/Malto-dextrins/Fructose/Lactic Acid	Glucose
	Alcohol
	Corn flour
	Corn oil
	Corn sugar
	Food starch—modified
	Sorbitol
	Vinegar
Legume	Acacia gum
	Arabic gum
	Carob
	Haraya gum
	Locust bean gum
	Tragacanth
Soy	Soy protein
	Garden or veggie burgers
	Hydrolyzed vegetable protein
	Lecithin
	Miso
	Modified food starch
	Soy concentrate
	Soya flour

Allergen	Ingredient Term
Soy (continued)	Soybean
	Soy cheese
	Soy milk
	Soy sauce
	Soy yogurt
	Tempeh
	Tofu
	TVP (textured vegetable protein)
	Vegetable protein concentrate
Wheat	Wheat
	All-purpose flour
	Bran
	Cake flour
	Farina, or Cream of Wheat
	Gluten flour
	Graham
	Graham flour
	Malt or cereal extract
	Modified food starch
	Pastry flour
	Semolina
	Wheat germ

Nutrition Resources

It is vital to have sound nutrition information when you need it. Sources can include magazines, newspapers, the Internet, or television. Your main concern should be having sources that are credible and trustworthy. Credible nutrition reports are careful with their wording and will not mislead you. Credible research should come from credible institutions, health professionals, reputable journals, and scientists. Before you take the nutritional advice of something you read or hear, consult a registered dietitian or other qualified nutrition expert or doctor. The following associations and Web sites will lead you to reliable nutrition information.

American Cancer Society
☎ 800-ACS-2345
🖱 www.cancer.org

American College of Gastroenterology (ACG)
4900 B South, 31st St.
Arlington, VA 22206
☎ 703-820-7400
🖱 www.acg.gi.org

American College of Sports Medicine
P.O. Box 1440
Indianapolis, IN 46206-1440
☎ 317-637-9200
🖱 www.acsm.org

American Council on Exercise
4851 Paramount Drive
San Diego, California 92123
☎ 800-825-3636
🖱 www.acefitness.com/

American Diabetes Association
ATTN: Customer Service
1701 North Beauregard Street
Alexandria, VA 22311
☎ 800-DIABETES (800-342-2383)
🖱 www.diabetes.org

American Dietetic Association
216 W. Jackson Blvd.
Chicago, IL 60606-6995
☎ 312-899-0040
🖱 www.eatright.org

American Dietetic Association's Market Place
🖱 www.eatright.com/catalog/consumer.html

American Heart Association
National Center
7272 Greenville Avenue
Dallas, TX 75231
☎ 800-AHA-USA-1 (800-242-8721)
🖱 www.americanheart.org

Celiac Disease Foundation
13251 Ventura Blvd., #1
Studio City, CA 91604
☎ 818-990-2354
🖱 www.celiac.org/

Consumer Nutrition Information Hotline
The American Dietetic Association
☎ 800-366-1655
🖱 hotline@eatright.org

Dietary Specialties
This company sells gluten-free foods
248 Sussex Tpk Unit C-2
Randolph, NJ 07869
📞 888-640-2800
✍ *www.dietspec.com/Default.html*

Food Allergy Network
Alletess Medical
216 Pleasant Street
Rockland, MA 02370
📞 800-225-5404
✍ *alletess@foodallergy.com*
✍ *www.foodallergy.com*

FDA (Food and Drug Administration)
5600 Fishers Lane
Rockville, MD 20857-0001
📞 888-INFO-FDA (1-888-463-6332)
✍ *www.fda.gov*

Food and Nutrition Information Center
10301 Baltimore Avenue
Beltsville, MD 20705-2351
📞 301-504-5719
✍ *fnic@nal.usda.gov*
✍ *www.nal.usda.gov/fnic/*

Health Finder
✍ *www.healthfinder.gov*

Institute of Medicine
The National Academies
2001 Wisconsin Avenue, N.W.
Washington, DC 20007
✍ *iomwww@nas.edu*
✍ *www.iom.edu/*

Kingsmill Food Company, Ltd.
This company sells gluten-free foods
1399 Kennedy Rd, Unit 17
Toronto, Ontario, Canada, M1P 2L6
📞 416-755-1124
✍ *www.kingsmillfoods.com*

National Eating Disorders Association
603 Stewart St., Suite 803
Seattle, WA 98101
📞 206-382-3587
✍ *info@NationalEatingDisorders.org*
✍ *www.nationaleatingdisorders.org*

National Institute of Diabetes and Digestive
and Kidney Disorders
31 Center Dr.
Bethesda, MD 20892
📞 301-496-3583
✍ *www.niddk.nih.gov*

National Institutes of Health
Bethesda, MD 20892
📞 301-496-4000
✍ *www.nih.gov*

North American Vegetarian Society
P.O. Box 72
Dolgeville, NY 13329
📞 518-568-7970
✍ *navs@telenet.net*
✍ *www.navs-online.org/*

Nutrition Action Health Letter
Center for Science in the Public Interest
1875 Connecticut Ave., N.W., Suite 300
Washington, D.C. 20009
📞 202-332-9110
✍ *cspi@cspinet.org*
✍ *www.cspinet.org*

United Soybean Board
16640 Chesterfield Grove Road
Suite 130
Chesterfield, MO 63005
📞 800-989-USB1 (800-989-8721)
✍ *info@talksoy.com*
✍ *www.unitedsoybean.org*
✍ *www.talksoy.com*
✍ *www.soybean.org*

U.S. Department of Health and Human Services
200 Independence Avenue, S.W.
Washington, D.C. 20201
☏ 877-696-6775
✉ HHS.Mail@hhs.gov
✉ www.dhhs.gov

The U.S. Soyfoods Directory
Published by: Stevens & Associates, Inc.
4816 North Pennsylvania Street
Indianapolis, IN 46205-1744
✉ info@soyfoods.com
✉ www.soyfoods.com

The Vegetarian Resource Group
P.O. Box 1463
Baltimore, MD 21203
☏ 410-366-8343
✉ vrg@vrg.org
✉ www.vrg.org

Tufts University Diet and Nutrition Letter
10 High Street, Suite 706
Boston, MA 02110
✉ healthletter@tufts.edu
✉ www.healthletter.tufts.edu

Vegan Action
P.O. Box 4288
Richmond, VA 23220
☏ 804-254-8346
✉ info@vegan.org
✉ www.vegan.org

Vegetarian Times
301 Concourse Blvd. Ste. 240 Hop
Glen Allen, VA 23059.
✉ www.vegetariantimes.com

Vegsource.com
✉ www.vegsource.com

Weight Control Information Network
✉ www.niddk.nih.gov/health/nutrit/nutrit.htm

Weight Loss for Life
✉ www.niddk.nih.gov/health/nutrit/pubs/wtloss/
wtloss.htm

Index

A

acesulfame-K, 152–153

acid reflux, during pregnancy, 227–228

Adequate Intake (AI), 73–74

after-school snack ideas, 203–204

alcoholic beverages
    breastfeeding and, 230
    cancer and, 259
    at college, 215–216
    consuming in moderation, 20
    exercise and, 284

allergies
    to breast milk, 188
    contrasted to food intolerance, 248
    diagnosing of, 250
    food label terms and, 291–292
    to milk, 39, 251
    to solid foods, 190, 194–196
    symptoms of, 248–250
    treatment of, 250–251
    see also lactose intolerance

amino acids, 60–61

anaphylactic reaction, 249–250

anemia, 81–82, 96, 189

anorexia nervosa, 210–211, 242–243

anticoagulants, vitamin K and, 78

antioxidants, 32, 72
    vitamin E and, 77, 138–139

anxiety, caffeine and, 50

apple body shape, 5–6

artificial sweeteners, 144, 150–151
    acesulfame-K, 152–153
    aspartame, 151–152
    saccharin, 152
    safety of, 153–155
    sucralose, 153

ascorbic acid (vitamin C), 83–84, 224
    sources of, 84, 258, 289

aspartame, 151–152

athletes, protein and, 63. See also exercise

B

baking tips, 180–181

basal metabolic rate, 11–12

beans, see meat group

beta-carotene, 74–76, 223, 258

beverages, sugar in, 19–20. See also alcoholic beverages; soft drinks; water

binge eating disorders, 244–245

bioelectric impedance analysis (BIA), 7–8

biotin, 83

birth defects, 171, 222–223

blood pressure, high, 116–118, 260
    control of, 262
    food label health claims and, 171
    risk factors for, 261

blood sugar, see glucose

body composition, measuring, 6–9

body fat
    healthy range for, 6–9
    measuring of, 6–10
    see also weight issues

body mass index (BMI), 9–10, 288

body shape, health and, 5–6

"braising," defined, 182

bread, cereal, rice, pasta group, 26–28
    needed during pregnancy, 222

THE EVERYTHING SERIES!

BUSINESS

Everything® **Business Planning Book**
Everything® **Coaching and Mentoring Book**
Everything® **Fundraising Book**
Everything® **Home-Based Business Book**
Everything® **Leadership Book**
Everything® **Managing People Book**
Everything® **Network Marketing Book**
Everything® **Online Business Book**
Everything® **Project Management Book**
Everything® **Selling Book**
Everything® **Start Your Own Business Book**
Everything® **Time Management Book**

COMPUTERS

Everything® **Build Your Own Home Page Book**
Everything® **Computer Book**
Everything® **Internet Book**
Everything® **Microsoft® Word 2000 Book**

COOKBOOKS

Everything® **Barbecue Cookbook**
Everything® **Bartender's Book, $9.95**
Everything® **Chinese Cookbook**
Everything® **Chocolate Cookbook**
Everything® **Cookbook**
Everything® **Dessert Cookbook**
Everything® **Diabetes Cookbook**
Everything® **Indian Cookbook**
Everything® **Low-Carb Cookbook**
Everything® **Low-Fat High-Flavor Cookbook**

Everything® **Low-Salt Cookbook**
Everything® **Mediterranean Cookbook**
Everything® **Mexican Cookbook**
Everything® **One-Pot Cookbook**
Everything® **Pasta Book**
Everything® **Quick Meals Cookbook**
Everything® **Slow Cooker Cookbook**
Everything® **Soup Cookbook**
Everything® **Thai Cookbook**
Everything® **Vegetarian Cookbook**
Everything® **Wine Book**

HEALTH

Everything® **Alzheimer's Book**
Everything® **Anti-Aging Book**
Everything® **Diabetes Book**
Everything® **Dieting Book**
Everything® **Herbal Remedies Book**
Everything® **Hypnosis Book**
Everything® **Massage Book**
Everything® **Menopause Book**
Everything® **Nutrition Book**
Everything® **Reflexology Book**
Everything® **Reiki Book**
Everything® **Stress Management Book**
Everything® **Vitamins, Minerals, and Nutritional Supplements Book**

HISTORY

Everything® **American Government Book**
Everything® **American History Book**
Everything® **Civil War Book**
Everything® **Irish History & Heritage Book**

Everything® **Mafia Book**
Everything® **Middle East Book**
Everything® **World War II Book**

HOBBIES & GAMES

Everything® **Bridge Book**
Everything® **Candlemaking Book**
Everything® **Casino Gambling Book**
Everything® **Chess Basics Book**
Everything® **Collectibles Book**
Everything® **Crossword and Puzzle Book**
Everything® **Digital Photography Book**
Everything® **Easy Crosswords Book**
Everything® **Family Tree Book**
Everything® **Games Book**
Everything® **Knitting Book**
Everything® **Magic Book**
Everything® **Motorcycle Book**
Everything® **Online Genealogy Book**
Everything® **Photography Book**
Everything® **Pool & Billiards Book**
Everything® **Quilting Book**
Everything® **Scrapbooking Book**
Everything® **Sewing Book**
Everything® **Soapmaking Book**

HOME IMPROVEMENT

Everything® **Feng Shui Book**
Everything® **Feng Shui Decluttering Book, $9.95 ($15.95 CAN)**
Everything® **Fix-It Book**
Everything® **Gardening Book**
Everything® **Homebuilding Book**

All Everything® books are priced at $12.95 or $14.95, unless otherwise stated. Prices subject to change without notice.
Canadian prices range from $11.95–$31.95, and are subject to change without notice.

Everything® **Home Decorating Book**
Everything® **Landscaping Book**
Everything® **Lawn Care Book**
Everything® **Organize Your Home Book**

EVERYTHING® KIDS' BOOKS

All titles are $6.95
Everything® **Kids' Baseball Book, 3rd Ed. ($10.95 CAN)**
Everything® **Kids' Bible Trivia Book ($10.95 CAN)**
Everything® **Kids' Bugs Book ($10.95 CAN)**
Everything® **Kids' Christmas Puzzle & Activity Book ($10.95 CAN)**
Everything® **Kids' Cookbook ($10.95 CAN)**
Everything® **Kids' Halloween Puzzle & Activity Book ($10.95 CAN)**
Everything® **Kids' Joke Book ($10.95 CAN)**
Everything® **Kids' Math Puzzles Book ($10.95 CAN)**
Everything® **Kids' Mazes Book ($10.95 CAN)**
Everything® **Kids' Money Book ($11.95 CAN)**
Everything® **Kids' Monsters Book ($10.95 CAN)**
Everything® **Kids' Nature Book ($11.95 CAN)**
Everything® **Kids' Puzzle Book ($10.95 CAN)**
Everything® **Kids' Riddles & Brain Teasers Book ($10.95 CAN)**
Everything® **Kids' Science Experiments Book ($10.95 CAN)**
Everything® **Kids' Soccer Book ($10.95 CAN)**
Everything® **Kids' Travel Activity Book ($10.95 CAN)**

KIDS' STORY BOOKS

Everything® **Bedtime Story Book**
Everything® **Bible Stories Book**
Everything® **Fairy Tales Book**
Everything® **Mother Goose Book**

LANGUAGE

Everything® **Inglés Book**
Everything® **Learning French Book**
Everything® **Learning German Book**
Everything® **Learning Italian Book**
Everything® **Learning Latin Book**
Everything® **Learning Spanish Book**
Everything® **Sign Language Book**
Everything® **Spanish Phrase Book, $9.95 ($15.95 CAN)**

MUSIC

Everything® **Drums Book (with CD), $19.95 ($31.95 CAN)**
Everything® **Guitar Book**
Everything® **Playing Piano and Keyboards Book**
Everything® **Rock & Blues Guitar Book (with CD), $19.95 ($31.95 CAN)**
Everything® **Songwriting Book**

NEW AGE

Everything® **Astrology Book**
Everything® **Divining the Future Book**
Everything® **Dreams Book**
Everything® **Ghost Book**
Everything® **Love Signs Book, $9.95 ($15.95 CAN)**
Everything® **Meditation Book**
Everything® **Numerology Book**
Everything® **Palmistry Book**
Everything® **Psychic Book**
Everything® **Spells & Charms Book**
Everything® **Tarot Book**
Everything® **Wicca and Witchcraft Book**

PARENTING

Everything® **Baby Names Book**
Everything® **Baby Shower Book**
Everything® **Baby's First Food Book**
Everything® **Baby's First Year Book**
Everything® **Breastfeeding Book**

Everything® **Father-to-Be Book**
Everything® **Get Ready for Baby Book**
Everything® **Getting Pregnant Book**
Everything® **Homeschooling Book**
Everything® **Parent's Guide to Children with Autism**
Everything® **Parent's Guide to Positive Discipline**
Everything® **Parent's Guide to Raising a Successful Child**
Everything® **Parenting a Teenager Book**
Everything® **Potty Training Book, $9.95 ($15.95 CAN)**
Everything® **Pregnancy Book, 2nd Ed.**
Everything® **Pregnancy Fitness Book**
Everything® **Pregnancy Organizer, $15.00 ($22.95 CAN)**
Everything® **Toddler Book**
Everything® **Tween Book**

PERSONAL FINANCE

Everything® **Budgeting Book**
Everything® **Get Out of Debt Book**
Everything® **Get Rich Book**
Everything® **Homebuying Book, 2nd Ed.**
Everything® **Homeselling Book**
Everything® **Investing Book**
Everything® **Money Book**
Everything® **Mutual Funds Book**
Everything® **Online Investing Book**
Everything® **Personal Finance Book**
Everything® **Personal Finance in Your 20s & 30s Book**
Everything® **Wills & Estate Planning Book**

PETS

Everything® **Cat Book**
Everything® **Dog Book**
Everything® **Dog Training and Tricks Book**
Everything® **Golden Retriever Book**
Everything® **Horse Book**
Everything® **Labrador Retriever Book**
Everything® **Puppy Book**
Everything® **Tropical Fish Book**

All Everything® books are priced at $12.95 or $14.95, unless otherwise stated. Prices subject to change without notice.
Canadian prices range from $11.95–$31.95, and are subject to change without notice.

REFERENCE

Everything® **Astronomy Book**
Everything® **Car Care Book**
Everything® **Christmas Book, $15.00**
  ($21.95 CAN)
Everything® **Classical Mythology Book**
Everything® **Einstein Book**
Everything® **Etiquette Book**
Everything® **Great Thinkers Book**
Everything® **Philosophy Book**
Everything® **Psychology Book**
Everything® **Shakespeare Book**
Everything® **Tall Tales, Legends, &**
  Other Outrageous
  Lies Book
Everything® **Toasts Book**
Everything® **Trivia Book**
Everything® **Weather Book**

RELIGION

Everything® **Angels Book**
Everything® **Bible Book**
Everything® **Buddhism Book**
Everything® **Catholicism Book**
Everything® **Christianity Book**
Everything® **Jewish History &**
  Heritage Book
Everything® **Judaism Book**
Everything® **Prayer Book**
Everything® **Saints Book**
Everything® **Understanding Islam**
  Book
Everything® **World's Religions Book**
Everything® **Zen Book**

SCHOOL & CAREERS

Everything® **After College Book**
Everything® **Alternative Careers Book**
Everything® **College Survival Book**
Everything® **Cover Letter Book**
Everything® **Get-a-Job Book**
Everything® **Hot Careers Book**

Everything® **Job Interview Book**
Everything® **New Teacher Book**
Everything® **Online Job Search Book**
Everything® **Resume Book, 2nd Ed.**
Everything® **Study Book**

SELF-HELP/ RELATIONSHIPS

Everything® **Dating Book**
Everything® **Divorce Book**
Everything® **Great Marriage Book**
Everything® **Great Sex Book**
Everything® **Kama Sutra Book**
Everything® **Romance Book**
Everything® **Self-Esteem Book**
Everything® **Success Book**

SPORTS & FITNESS

Everything® **Body Shaping Book**
Everything® **Fishing Book**
Everything® **Fly-Fishing Book**
Everything® **Golf Book**
Everything® **Golf Instruction Book**
Everything® **Knots Book**
Everything® **Pilates Book**
Everything® **Running Book**
Everything® **Sailing Book, 2nd Ed.**
Everything® **T'ai Chi and QiGong Book**
Everything® **Total Fitness Book**
Everything® **Weight Training Book**
Everything® **Yoga Book**

TRAVEL

Everything® **Family Guide to Hawaii**
Everything® **Guide to Las Vegas**
Everything® **Guide to New England**
Everything® **Guide to New York City**
Everything® **Guide to Washington D.C.**
Everything® **Travel Guide to The**
  Disneyland Resort®,
  California Adventure®,

Universal Studios®, **and**
  the Anaheim Area
Everything® **Travel Guide to the Walt**
  Disney World Resort®,
  Universal Studios®, and
  Greater Orlando, 3rd Ed.

WEDDINGS

Everything® **Bachelorette Party Book,**
  $9.95 ($15.95 CAN)
Everything® **Bridesmaid Book, $9.95**
  ($15.95 CAN)
Everything® **Creative Wedding Ideas**
  Book
Everything® **Elopement Book, $9.95**
  ($15.95 CAN)
Everything® **Groom Book**
Everything® **Jewish Wedding Book**
Everything® **Wedding Book, 2nd Ed.**
Everything® **Wedding Checklist,**
  $7.95 ($11.95 CAN)
Everything® **Wedding Etiquette Book,**
  $7.95 ($11.95 CAN)
Everything® **Wedding Organizer,**
  $15.00 ($22.95 CAN)
Everything® **Wedding Shower Book,**
  $7.95 ($12.95 CAN)
Everything® **Wedding Vows Book,**
  $7.95 ($11.95 CAN)
Everything® **Weddings on a Budget**
  Book, $9.95 ($15.95 CAN)

WRITING

Everything® **Creative Writing Book**
Everything® **Get Published Book**
Everything® **Grammar and Style Book**
Everything® **Grant Writing Book**
Everything® **Guide to Writing**
  Children's Books
Everything® **Screenwriting Book**
Everything® **Writing Well Book**

Available wherever books are sold!
To order, call 800-872-5627, or visit us at everything.com